Thomas S. Szasz, M.D., was born in Budapest, Hungary, in 1920. He went to the United States at the age of eighteen, and attended the University of Cincinnati, receiving his A.B. in 1941 with honours in Physics. He received his M.D. from the University of Cincinnati's College of Medicine in 1944. Dr Szasz subsequently served his psychiatric residency at the University of Chicago Clinics from 1946 to 1948 and underwent psychoanalytic training at the Chicago Institute for Psychoanalysis, 1947–50.

Dr Szasz received his Certification in Psychiatry from the American Board of Psychiatry and Neurology in 1951, and became a staff member of the Chicago Institute for Psychoanalysis. Since 1956, he has been Professor of Psychiatry at the Upstate Medical Center of the State University of New York in Syracuse, New York. He is the author of numerous books including *Pain and Pleasure, Law, Liberty and Psychiatry, Ideology and Insanity* and, most recently, *The Manufacture of Madness*. He is a contributor to books, journals, and symposia on philosophical, legal, psychiatric, and psychoanalytic subjects.

THOMAS S. SZASZ

The Myth of Mental Illness

Foundations of a Theory of Personal Conduct

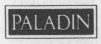

Granada Publishing

Paladin Books
Granada Publishing Ltd
8 Grafton Street, London W1X 3LA

Published by Paladin Books 1972
Reprinted 1972, 1973, 1975, 1977, 1981, 1984

First published in Great Britain by
Secker & Warburg Ltd 1962

Copyright © Hoeber Medical Division
Harper & Row Publishers Inc 1961

ISBN 0-586-08087-2

Made and printed in Great Britain by
Hazell Watson & Viney Limited,
Aylesbury, Bucks

Set in Linotype Pilgrim

To my wife, Rosine

Science must begin with myths, and with the criticism of myths.

Karl R. Popper (1957, p. 177)

Contents

Part IV. Game-model Analysis of Behaviour

Preface to the Paladin Edition

Every book is, inevitably, part autobiography. I started work on this book in 1954, when, having been called to active duty in the navy, I was relieved of the burdens of a full-time psychoanalytic practice and could turn my energies to putting on paper something of what had long been in my mind. The first publisher to whom I submitted the manuscript of *The Myth of Mental Illness*, in 1957 or 1958 I think, deliberated about it at length and then rejected it. I next sent it to Mr Paul Hoeber, then the director of the medical division of Harper & Brothers (now Harper & Row, Publishers), to whom I am grateful for publishing a book which, especially then, must have seemed to fly in the face of nearly everything that was known about psychiatry and psychoanalysis.

Within a year of its publication, the Commissioner of the New York State Department of Mental Hygiene demanded, in a letter citing specifically *The Myth of Mental Illness*, that I be dismissed from my university position because I did not 'believe' in mental illness. Neither the details of that affair nor the other consequences of my publishing this book belong in this Preface. Suffice it to say that much has happened to me since. And perhaps much, in part because of this book, has happened to psychiatry also.

Obviously, then, were I to write this book today I would write it differently. But I am, on the whole, still quite satisfied with the original work. However, the original version of *The Myth of Mental Illness* now appears to me unnecessarily detailed in the developments of its thesis, and overdocumented in its bibliography. I decided, therefore, that for this new Paladin edition I would eliminate everything that does not bear directly on its main themes. At the same time I rejected the temptation to add any fresh material (except for this Preface and a brief new

Summary), partly because, once begun, such rewriting would have been difficult to control, and partly because, in several of my books published since 1961, I have elaborated on the ideas first presented here.

The problems to which I address myself in this book are easy to state but, because of the powerful cultural and economic pressures that define the 'correct' answers to them, are difficult to clarify. They have to do with such questions as: What is disease? What are the ostensible and actual tasks of the physician? What is mental illness? Who defines what constitutes illness, diagnosis, treatment? Who controls the vocabulary of medicine and psychiatry, and the powers of physician-psychiatrist and citizen-patient? Has a person the right to call himself sick? Has a physician the right to call a person mentally sick? What is the difference between a person complaining of pain and calling himself sick? Or between a physician complaining of a person's misbehaviour and calling him a mentally sick patient? Without attempting to answer these questions or trying to anticipate the contents of this book, let me show briefly the sort of reasoning I bring to it.

When a person claims to be ill, he usually means, firstly, that he suffers, or believes he suffers, from an abnormality or mal-functioning of his body; and secondly, that he wants, or is at least willing to accept, medical help for it. If the first of these conditions is absent, we do not consider the person to be physically ill; if the second is absent, we do not consider him to be a medical patient. For the practice of modern Western medicine rests on the *scientific* premise that the physician's task is to diagnose and treat disorders of the human body, and on the *ethical* premise that he can carry out these services only with the consent of his patient.

To understand psychiatry, we must also understand the concept of mental illness, which arises in part from the fact that it is possible for a person to act *as if* he were sick without actually having a bodily illness. How should we deal with such a person? Should we treat him *as if* he were not ill, or *as if* he were? Today, it is considered shamefully uncivilized and naïvely unscientific to treat him as if he were not, everyone regarding such a person as *obviously* sick, that is, as 'mentally sick'. I believe this is a serious error. I hold that mental illness is a metaphorical disease; that, in other words, bodily illness stands in the same relation to mental illness as a defective television receiver stands to an objectionable television programme. To be sure, the word 'sick' is often used metaphorically. We call jokes 'sick', economies 'sick', sometimes even the whole world 'sick' – but only when we call minds 'sick' do we systematically mistake metaphor for fact; and send for the doctor to 'cure' the 'illness'. It's as if a television viewer were to send for a TV repairman because he disapproves of the programme he is watching.

Furthermore, just as it is possible for a person to define himself as sick without having a bodily illness, so it is also possible for a physician to define as 'sick' a person who feels perfectly well and wants no medical help, and then act *as if* he were a therapist trying to cure his 'patient's' disease. How should we react to such a physician? Should we treat him *as if* he were a malevolent meddler or a benevolent healer? Today, it is considered quite unscientific and uncivilized to adopt the former posture, everyone (except the victim, and sometimes even he, himself) regarding such a physician as obviously a therapist, that is, a psychiatric therapist. I believe this is a serious error. I hold that psychiatric interventions are directed at moral, not medical, problems; in other words, that psychiatric help sought by the client stands in the same relation to psychiatric intervention imposed on him as religious beliefs voluntarily professed stand to such beliefs imposed by force.

It is widely believed that mental illness is a type of disease, and that psychiatry is a branch of medicine; and yet, whereas people readily think of and call themselves 'sick', they rarely think of and call themselves 'mentally sick'. The reason for this, as I shall try to show, is really quite simple: a person might feel sad or elated, insignificant or grandiose, suicidal or homicidal, and so forth; he is, however, not likely to categorize himself as mentally ill or insane; that he is, is more likely to be suggested by someone else. This, then, is why bodily diseases are characteristically treated with the consent of the patient, while mental diseases are characteristically treated without his consent. (Individuals who nowadays seek private psychoanalytic or psychotherapeutic help do not, as a rule, consider themselves either 'sick' or 'mentally sick', but rather view their difficulties as problems in living and the help they receive as a type of counselling.) In short, while medical diagnoses are the names of genuine diseases, psychiatric diagnoses are stigmatizing labels.

Such considerations generate two diametrically opposite points of view about mental illness and psychiatry: according to the one, mental illness is like any other illness, and psychiatric treatment, whether voluntary or not, is like any other treatment; according to the other, mental illness is a myth, psychiatric intervention is a type of social action, and involuntary psychiatric therapy is not treatment but torture. This book attempts to demonstrate the fallacy of the former view, and the validity of the latter.

My brother, Dr George Szasz, and my secretary, Mrs Margaret Bassett, have been of immense help in preparing this new, abbreviated version of *The Myth of Mental Illness*. I am also grateful to Mr Sonny Mehta of Paladin Books for making this work once again available to the English-speaking public outside the United States.

Thomas S. Szasz, M.D.
Syracuse, New York
1 January 1972

Preface to the American Edition

I became interested in writing this book approximately ten years ago when, having become established as a psychiatrist, I became increasingly impressed by the vague, capricious, and generally unsatisfactory character of the widely used concept of mental illness and its corollaries, diagnosis, prognosis, and treatment. It seemed to me that although the notion of mental illness made good *historical* sense – stemming as it does from the historical identity of medicine and psychiatry – it made no *rational* sense. Mental illness might have been a useful concept in the nineteenth century; today it is scientifically worthless and socially harmful.

Although dissatisfaction with the medical basis and conceptual framework of psychiatry is not of recent origin, little has been done to make the problem explicit, and even less to remedy it. In psychiatric circles it is almost indelicate to ask: What is mental illness? In non-psychiatric circles mental illness all too often is considered to be whatever psychiatrists say it is. The answer to the question, Who is mentally ill? thus becomes: Those who are confined in mental hospitals or who consult psychiatrists in their private offices.

Perhaps these answers sound silly. If they do, it is because they are silly. However, it is not easy to give better answers without going to a good deal of trouble, firstly, by asking other questions, such as, Is mental illness an illness?, and secondly, by resetting one's goals from understanding mental illness to understanding human beings.

The need to re-examine the problem of mental illness is both timely and pressing. There is confusion, dissatisfaction, and tension in our society concerning psychiatric, psychological, and social issues. Mental illness is said to be the nation's number one health problem. The statistics marshalled to prove this contention are impressive: more than half a million hospital beds for mental patients, and seventeen million persons allegedly suffering from some degree of mental illness.

The concept of mental illness is freely used in all the major news media – the newspapers, radio, and television. Sometimes famous persons are said to be mentally ill – for example, Adolf Hitler, Ezra Pound, Earl Long. At other times the label is attached to the most lowly and unfortunate members of society, especially if they are accused of a crime.

The popularity of psychotherapy, and people's alleged need for it, is rapidly increasing. At the same time it is impossible to answer the question, What is psychotherapy? The term 'psychotherapy' encompasses nearly everything that people do in the company of one another. Psychoanalysis, group psychotherapy, religious counselling, rehabilitation of prisoners, and many other activities, all are called 'psychotherapy'.

This book was written in an effort to dispel the perplexities mentioned, and thereby to clear the psychiatric air. Part I is devoted to laying bare the sociohistorical and epistemological roots of the modern concept of mental illness. The question, What *is* mental illness? is shown to be inextricably tied to the question, What do psychiatrists *do*? My first task, accordingly, is to present an essentially 'destructive' analysis of the concept of mental illness and of psychiatry as a pseudo-medical enterprise. I believe that such 'destruction', like tearing down old buildings, is necessary if we are to construct a new, more habitable edifice for the study of man.

Since it is difficult to scrap one conceptual model without having another with which to replace it, I had to search for a new point of view. My second aim, then, is to offer a 'constructive' synthesis of the knowledge which I have found useful for filling the gap left by casting off the myth of mental illness. Parts II, III, and IV are devoted to presenting a systematic theory of personal conduct, based partly on materials culled from psychiatry, psychoanalysis, and other disciplines, and partly on my own observations and ideas. The omission from psychiatric theories of moral issues and normative standards, as explicitly stated goals and rules of conduct, has divorced psychiatry from precisely that reality which it has tried to describe and explain.

I have endeavoured to correct this defect by means of a game-theory of human living, which enables us to combine ethical, political, religious, and social considerations with the more traditional concerns of medicine and psychiatry.

In sum, then, this is not a book *on* psychiatry. It is a book *about* psychiatry – inquiring into what psychiatrists and patients have done, and continue to do, with and to one another. It is also a book about human nature, but more particularly about human conduct – since in it observations and hypotheses are offered concerning how people live.

Introduction

Sooner or later every scientific enterprise comes to a fork in the road. Scientists must then decide which of two paths to follow. The dilemma that must be faced is: how shall we conceive of what we do? Should we think of it in terms of *substantives* and *entities* – for example, elements, compounds, living things, mental illnesses, and so forth? Or should we think of it in terms of *processes* and *activities* – for example, Brownian movement, oxidation, or communication? These two modes of conceptualization represent a developmental sequence in the evolution of scientific thought. Entity-thinking has always preceded process-thinking. Physics, chemistry, and certain branches of biology have long ago supplemented substantive conceptualizations by process-theories. Psychiatry has not.

Scope and Methods of the Study

I submit that the traditional definition of psychiatry, which is still in vogue, places it alongside such things as alchemy and astrology, and commits it to the category of pseudo-science. Psychiatry is said to be a medical speciality concerned with the study and treatment of mental illness. Similarly, astrology was the study of the influence of planetary movements and positions on human behaviour and destiny. These are typical instances of defining a science by specifying its subject-matter. But these definitions completely disregard method and rely instead on false substantives. The activities of alchemists and astrologers – in contrast to the activities of chemists and astronomers – were not bound by publicly disclosed methods of observation and inference. Psychiatrists, likewise, have persistently avoided disclosing fully and publicly what they do. Indeed, whether as therapists or theorists they may do virtually anything and still be considered psychiatrists. Thus, the behaviour of a particular psychiatrist – as a member of the category 'psychiatrist' – may be that of a physician, policeman, clergyman, friend, counsellor, teacher, psychoanalyst, or all manner of combinations of these. He is a psychiatrist so long as he claims that he is oriented towards the problem of mental illness and health. But suppose, for a moment, that there is no such thing as mental illness and health. Suppose, further, that these words refer to nothing more substantial or real than the astrological conception of planetary influences on human conduct. What then?

Methods of Observation and Action in Psychiatry

Psychiatry stands at the crossroads. Thus far, thinking in terms of substantives – for example, neurosis, disease, treatment – has been the rule. The question is: shall we continue along the same road or branch off in the direction of process-thinking? Viewed in this light, my efforts in this study are directed, firstly, *at demolishing some of the major false substantives of contemporary psychiatric thought*, and, secondly, *at laying the foundations for a process-theory of personal conduct*.

Discrepancies between what people say they do and what they actually do are encountered in all walks of life, science included. The principle of operationism, made into a systematic philosophy of science by Bridgman (1936), was succinctly formulated by Einstein (1933) in connection with exactly this discrepancy in physics:

If you want to find out anything from the theoretical physicists about the methods they use, I advise you to stick closely to one principle: Don't listen to their words, fix your attention on their deeds. (p. 30)

Surely there is no reason to assume that this principle is any less valid for understanding the methods – and hence the nature and subject – of psychiatry.

Briefly stated, an operational definition of a concept is one that relates it to actual 'operations'. A physical concept is defined by physical operations, such as measurements of time, temperature, distance, and so forth. Operational definitions may be contrasted with idealistic definitions, the latter being exemplified by the classic, pre-Einsteinian notions of time, space, and mass. Similarly, a psychological or sociological concept, defined operationally, relates to psychological or sociological observations or measurements. In contrast, many psychosocial concepts are defined on the basis of the investigator's self-proclaimed intentions or values. The majority of present-day psychiatric concepts belong in the latter category.

The answer to the question: What do psychiatrists do? depends, therefore, on the kind of psychiatrist one has in mind. He might be any of the following (the list is not necessarily complete): one who physically examines patients, administers drugs and electric shock treatments, signs commitment papers, examines criminals and testifies concerning them in courts, or, most commonly, perhaps, listens and talks to persons. In this book I shall be concerned mainly with psychiatry as a special discipline whose method is, rather derisively but nevertheless quite correctly, often spoken of as 'only talking'. If the word 'only' is disregarded as gratuitous condemnation, and if the meaning of 'talking' is enlarged to encompass communications of all kinds, we arrive at the formulation of a basic method of psychiatry to which surprisingly few psychiatrists really subscribe. In fact there is a split, perhaps even an unbridgeable gap, between what most psychotherapists and psychoanalysts *do* in practice and what they *say* about it. What they do, of course, is to communicate with patients by means of language, non-verbal signs, and rules. Further, they analyse, by means of verbal symbols, the communicative interactions which they observe and in which they themselves engage. This, I believe, correctly describes the actual operations of psychoanalysis and psychosocially oriented psychiatry. But what do these psychiatrists tell themselves and others concerning their work? They talk as if they were physicians, physiologists, biologists, or even physicists! We hear about 'sick patients', 'instincts' and 'endocrine functions', and of course 'libido' and 'psychic energies', both 'free' and 'bound'. While the need for clarity in regard to method and language is no longer a new idea among scientists, it requires re-emphasis in our field.

Psychiatry, using the methods of communication analysis, has much in common with the sciences concerned with the study of languages and communicative behaviour. In spite of this connection between psychiatry and such disciplines as symbolic logic, semiotic,[1] and sociology, problems of mental health continue to be cast in the traditional framework of medicine. The conceptual scaffolding of medicine, on the other hand, rests on the principles of physics and chemistry. This is entirely reasonable, for it has been, and continues to be, the task of medicine to study – and if necessary to alter – the physicochemical structure and function of the human body. Man's sign-using behaviour, however, does not lend itself to exploration and understanding in these terms.

The distinction between psychology and physics is, of course, a familiar one. The differences, however, are not usually taken seriously enough. The lack of commitment to psychology as a legitimate science is revealed by some scientists' outspoken expectation that in the end all scientific observations and statements will be phrased in a mathematico-physical idiom. More specifically, in the language of psychiatry and psychoanalysis infidelity to subject and method is expressed in the persistent imitation of medicine. Thus we continue to speak of and presumably believe in such notions as 'psychopathology' and 'psychotherapy'. This, at least, is the manifest state of our discipline. At the same time, ideas concerning object relationships and communications have gained greater acceptance, especially in recent decades. But a science can be no better than its linguistic apparatus permits. Hence our continued reliance on such notions as 'neurosis', 'psychosis', 'emotional illness', 'psychoanalytic treatment', and so forth cannot be lightly dismissed. We remain shackled to a scientifically outmoded conceptual framework and its terminology. We cannot, however, for ever hold fast to and profit from the morally judgemental and socially manipulative character of our traditional psychiatric and psychoanalytic vocabulary without paying a price for it. I believe that we are in danger of purchasing superiority and power over non-psychiatrists and patients at the cost of scientific self-sterilization and hence ultimate professional self-destruction.

[1] The term 'semiotic' designates the *science of signs* (Morris, 1946, 1955).

The issues of historical constancy and predictability are of the utmost importance for all of psychiatry. Questions such as whether hysteria was 'always the same disease' revolve around it, as does also the question of whether a psychotherapist can 'predict' whether Mr X will be happy in marriage with Miss Y. It is implicit in traditional psychoanalytic thought that prediction is a legitimate concern of this science. One often hears, nowadays, how prediction ought to be used to 'validate' psychoanalytic hypotheses. I believe we should have serious reservations concerning such preoccupations with controlling and predicting psychosocial occurrences.

The psychoanalytic theory of man was fashioned after the causal-deterministic model of classical physics. The errors of this transposition have been amply documented in recent years (e.g. Gregory, 1953). I wish to call attention here to that application of the principle of physical determinism to human affairs which Popper (1944–5) aptly termed 'historicism'. Examination of much of modern psychiatric thought discloses the fundamental role of antecedent historical events as alleged *determinants* of subsequent behaviour. The psychoanalytic theory of behaviour is, therefore, a species of historicism. As long as this type of explanation is considered satisfactory, there is no need for other types of explanations, such as will be presented in this book. It should be kept in mind, moreover, that historicist theories of behaviour preclude explanations of valuation, choice, and responsibility in human affairs.

Briefly stated, historicism is a doctrine according to which historical prediction is essentially no different from physical prediction. Historical events are viewed as fully determined by their antecedents, just as physical events are by theirs. The prediction of future events is, therefore, possible, at least in principle. In practice, prediction is considered to be limited by the extent to which past and present conditions can be accurately determined. In so far as these can be adequately ascertained, successful prediction is assured.

Popper's models of historicist social thinkers are Plato, Nietzsche, Marx, and the modern totalitarian dictators and their apologists. According to historicist doctrine the future is irrevocably determined by the past: 'Every version of historicism expresses the feeling of being swept into the future by irresistible forces' (Popper, 1944–5, p. 160). Compare this with Freud's thesis that human conduct is determined by 'unconscious forces' which, in turn, are the results of instinctual drives and early experiences. The crucial similarity between Marxism and classical psychoanalysis thus lies in the selection of a single type of antecedent cause as sufficient explanation of virtually all subsequent human events: in Marxism, the 'causes' are economic conditions; in psychoanalysis, family-historical (so-called genetic-psychological) circumstances. Paradoxically, therapy is based on the expectation that reason and understanding might help to mitigate the otherwise irresistible forces of historicism. But whether the past is, in fact, as powerful a determinant of future human actions as it is of future physical events is a moot question. It is by no means the established fact that Freud claimed it was. Yet, this unsupported – and, I think, false – theory of personal conduct has become widely accepted in our day. It has even received legal authentication in certain criminal statutes that recognize some types of actions as the results of 'mental illness'.

The principal basis for the failure of historicism is that, in the social sciences, we are faced with a full and complicated interaction between observer and observed. Specifically, the prediction of a social event itself may cause it to occur or may lead to its prevention. The so-called self-fulfilling prophecy – in which the predictor helps bring about the predicted event – exemplifies the difficulties with which prediction in the social sphere is fraught. All this is not intended to deny or minimize the effects and significance of past experiences – that is, of historical antecedents – on subsequent human performances. This process, however, must be conceptualized and understood not in terms of antecedent 'causes' and subsequent 'effects', but rather in terms of modifications in the entire organization and functioning of the subject acted upon.

In view of the rather obvious empirical and logical inadequacies of historicist theories, one may ask: what is the value of subscribing to an historicist position? In addition to providing a painstaking refutation of historicism, Popper suggested an explanation of why many people adhere to it:

It really looks as if *historicists were trying to compensate themselves for the loss of an unchanging* world by clinging to the belief that *change can be foreseen* because it is ruled by an *unchanging law*. ([Italics added] p. 161)

Freud (1927) proposed a similar explanation for why men believe in religion, attributing it to man's inability to tolerate the loss of the familiar world of childhood, symbolized by the protective father. Thus, a 'father in heaven' and a replica of the protective childhood game are created to replace the father and the family lost in the here-and-now. The difference between religion and political historicism, from this point of view, is only in the specific identities of the 'protectors': they are God and the theologians, in the first instance; whereas, in the second, they are the modern totalitarian leaders and their apologists.

It is especially important to emphasize, therefore, that although Freud criticized organized religion for the infantilism that it is, he failed to apprehend the social characteristics of the 'closed society' and the psychological characteristics of its loyal supporters. The paradox that is psychoanalysis – consisting on the one hand of an historicist theory, and on the other of an anti-historicist therapy – thus came into being. Whatever the reasons – and many have been suggested – Freud adopted and promoted a biopsychological world view embodying the principle of constancy and resting squarely on it. We may assume that historicism had the same function for him, and for those who joined with him in the precarious early psychoanalytic movement, as it had for others: it provided a hidden source of comfort against the threat of unforeseen and unpredictable change. This interpretation is consonant with the current use of psychoanalysis and 'dynamic psychiatry' as means for obscuring and disguising moral and political conflicts as mere personal problems.

What, then, can we say about the relationship between psychosocial and physical laws? The two are not similar. Psychosocial antecedents do not 'cause' human sign-using behaviour in the same manner as physical antecedents 'cause' their effects. Furthermore, just as physical laws are relativistic with respect to mass, so psychological laws are relativistic with respect to social conditions. In short, *the laws of psychology cannot be formulated independently of the laws of sociology.*

Psychiatry and Ethics

From the point of view which will be presented here, *psychiatry, as a theoretical science, consists of the study of personal conduct* – of clarifying and explaining the kinds of games people play with each other; how they learned these games; why they like to play them; and so forth.[2] Actual behaviour is the raw data from which the rules of the game are inferred. From among the many different kinds of behaviour, the verbal form – or communication by means of conventional language – constitutes one of the central areas of interest for psychiatry. Thus it is in the structure of language games that the interests of linguistics, philosophy, psychiatry, and semiotic meet. Each of these disciplines has addressed itself to different aspects of the language game: linguistics to its structure, philosophy to its cognitive significa-tion, and psychiatry to its social usage.

I hope that this approach will effect a much-needed and long overdue *rapprochement* between psychiatry on the one hand and philosophy and ethics on the other. Questions such as How does man live? and How ought man to live? traditionally have been in the domains of philosophy, ethics, and religion. Until the latter part of the nineteenth century, psychology – and psy-chiatry, as a branch of it – was closely allied to philosophy and ethics. Since then, psychologists have considered themselves empirical scientists whose methods and theories are allegedly no different from those of the physicist or biologist. But in so far as psychologists address themselves to the two questions raised above, their methods and theories do differ from those of the natural scientists. Hence, psychiatrists cannot expect to solve moral problems by medical methods.

In sum, then, inasmuch as psychiatric theories seek to explain, and systems and psychotherapy to alter, human behaviour,

[2] A systematic analysis of personal conduct in terms of game-playing be-haviour will be presented in Part IV. The *model of games*, however, is used throughout the book. Although it is difficult to give a concise definition of the concept of game, game situations are characterized by a system of set roles and rules binding for all of the players.

statements concerning goals and values will be considered indispensable parts of theories of personal conduct and psychotherapy.

Hysteria as a Paradigm of Mental Illness

Modern psychiatry, if dated from Charcot's work on hysteria and hypnosis, is approximately one hundred years old. How did the study of so-called mental illnesses begin and develop? What economic, moral, political, and social forces helped to mould it into its present form? And, perhaps most important, what effect did medicine, and particularly the concept of bodily illness, have on the development of the concept of mental illness?

The strategy of this inquiry will be to answer these questions, using conversion hysteria as the historical paradigm of the sorts of phenomena to which the term 'mental illness' refers. Hysteria was selected for the following reasons.

Historically, it is the problem that captured the attention of the pioneer neuropsychiatrists (e.g., Charcot, Janet, Freud), and led to the gradual differentiation of neurology and psychiatry.

Logically, hysteria brings into focus the need to distinguish bodily illness from imitations of such illness. It presents the physician with the task of distinguishing the 'real' or genuine from the 'unreal' or false. The distinction between fact and facsimile – often apprehended as the distinction between object and sign, or between physics and psychology – remains the core-problem of contemporary psychiatric epistemology.

Psychosocially, conversion hysteria provides an excellent example of how so-called mental illness can best be conceptualized in terms of sign-using, rule-following, and game-playing, because (1) Hysteria is a form of non-verbal communication, making use of a special set of signs. (2) It is a system of rule-following behaviour, making special use of the rules of helplessness, illness, and coercion. (3) It is a game characterized by, among other things, the end-goals of domination and interpersonal control and by strategies of deceit.

Everything that will be said about hysteria pertains equally, in principle, to all other so-called mental illnesses and to personal conduct generally. The manifest diversity of mental illnesses –

for example, the differences between hysteria, obsessions, paranoia, schizophrenia, etc. – may be regarded as analogous to the manifest diversity characterizing different languages. But behind these phenomenological differences there are certain basic similarities. Within a particular family of languages, for instance the Indo-European, there are significant similarities of both structure and function. Thus, English and French have much in common, whereas both differ considerably from Hungarian. Similarly, hysterical picture language and dream language, both of which are composed largely of iconic signs, are closely related, and both differ significantly from a paranoid system which utilizes mainly conventional signs (that is, ordinary language). The characteristic configuration and impact of paranoid communications thus derives not from the peculiarity of the signs used but from the way everyday speech is used – that is, in an essentially object-seeking, persuasive-promotive manner.

Following an analysis of personal conduct as communication, I shall offer similar analyses of it in terms of rule-following and game-playing; and I shall show that of these three models, that of game-playing is the most comprehensive, as it contains the models of sign-using and rule-following.

In Part I, I shall examine how the modern concepts of hysteria and mental illness arose, developed, and now flourish. The sociohistorical contexts in which medicine, neurology, and later psychiatry were practised, as well as the logical foundation of basic medical and psychiatric concepts, will be the main areas of critical scrutiny.

This approach will require a careful examination of the problem of imitation, and of the logic of the relationship between the 'real' and the 'false', regardless of whether this distinction is encountered in medicine, psychiatry, or elsewhere. Since this distinction depends on human judgement, the criteria for making such judgements in medicine and psychiatry and the persons institutionally authorized to make them are of the greatest significance. The traditional medical criterion for distinguishing the genuine from the facsimile – that is, real illness from malingering – was the presence of *demonstrable change in bodily structure* as revealed by means of clinical examination of the patient, laboratory tests on bodily fluids, or post-mortem study of the cadaver.

Modern psychiatry began with the development of a new criterion for distinguishing real from false disease – namely, *alteration in bodily function* as revealed by the patient's complaints, or by observation of his behaviour. Conversion hysteria was thus the prototype of so-called *functional illness*. As paresis, for example, was considered a structural disease of the brain, so hysteria and mental illnesses generally were considered functional diseases of the same organ. So-called functional illnesses were thus placed in the same category as structural illnesses and were distinguished from imitated or faked illnesses by means of the criterion of *voluntary falsification*. Accordingly, hysteria, neurasthenia, obsessive-compulsive neurosis, depression, para-noia, and so forth were regarded as diseases that *happened* to people. Mentally sick persons did not 'will' their pathological behaviour and were therefore considered 'not responsible' for it. These mental diseases were henceforth contrasted with malinger-ing, which was the voluntary imitation of illness. Finally, in recent decades psychiatrists have claimed that malingering, too, is a form of mental illness. This poses a logical dilemma – the dilemma of the existence of an alleged entity called 'mental illness' which, even when deliberately counterfeited, is still 'mental illness'.

In addition to the empirical criteria for judging illness as real or false, the social position of the judge officially authorized to render such judgements is also of decisive significance. Some of the questions that arise in this connection are: What sorts of persons have the social power to make their judgements heard and to implement them? How do social class standing and the political structure of society affect the roles of the medical judge and of the potentially sick person? To answer these questions an inquiry into medical and psychiatric practices in different societies will be presented.

Foundations of a Theory of Personal Conduct

The Sign-Using Model of Behaviour

Although the view that psychiatry deals with the analysis of communications is no longer novel, the full implication of the idea that so-called mental illnesses are like languages, and unlike bodily diseases, has not been adequately articulated. Let us assume that the problem of hysteria resembles the problem of a person speaking a foreign language rather than that of a person having a bodily disease. We think of diseases as having 'causes', 'treatments', and 'cures'. However, if a person speaks a language other than our own, we do not look for the 'cause' of his peculiar linguistic behaviour: it would be foolish – and fruitless – to search for the 'aetiology' of speaking French. To understand such behaviour, we must think in terms of *learning* and *meaning*. Accordingly, we might conclude that speaking French is the result of living among people who speak French.

It follows, then, that if hysteria is regarded as a special form of communicative behaviour it is meaningless to inquire into its 'causes'. As with languages, we shall only be able to ask how hysteria was *learned* and what it *means*. This is exactly what Freud did with dreams. He regarded the dream as a language and proceeded to elucidate its structure and meanings.

If a so-called psychopathological phenomenon is more akin to a language than to an illness, it also follows that we cannot meaningfully talk about its 'treatment'. Although it is obvious that under certain circumstances it may be desirable for a person to change from one language to another – for example, to discontinue speaking French and begin speaking English – this change is not called a 'cure'. Speaking in terms of learning rather than in terms of aetiology permits one to acknowledge that among a diversity of communicative forms each has its own *raison d'être*, and that, because of the particular circumstances of the communicants, each is as 'valid' as any other.

I submit that hysteria – meaning thereby communication by means of bodily signs and complaints – constitutes a special form of sign-using behaviour. And I propose to call this type of communication *protolanguage*. This language has a twofold origin. Its first source is the human body, which is subject to disease and disability manifested by means of bodily signs (e.g. paralysis, convulsion, etc.) and bodily feelings (e.g. pain, fatigue, etc.). Its second source is culture and society, in particular the seemingly universal custom of making life easier, at least temporarily, for those who are ill. These two basic factors account for the development and use of the language of hysteria – *which is nothing other than the 'language of illness', employed either because another language has not been learned well enough, or because this language happens to be especially useful.* There may occur, of course, various combinations of these two reasons for using this language.

In Part II then, I will undertake a semiotical rather than a psychiatric or psychoanalytic analysis of hysteria. Firstly, I shall present a detailed examination of the structure and function of protolanguage. This will be followed by an exposition of the relations of protolanguage to the general class of non-discursive languages. And I will conclude with considerations of the problem of indirect communication – that is, an analysis of the structure and function of alluding, hinting, and implying.

The Rule-following Model of Behaviour

The concepts of rule-following and role-taking derive from the premise that personal conduct may be best studied by regarding man's 'mind' mainly as a product of his social environment. In other words, although there are certain biological invariants in behaviour, the precise pattern of human actions is determined largely by roles and rules. Accordingly, anthropology, ethics, and sociology are the basic sciences of human action, since they are concerned with values, goals, and rules of human behaviour.

With the introduction of the rule-following model as a frame of reference for hysteria and mental illness, two questions naturally arise: (1) What kind of rules are there, and how do they influence behaviour? (2) Which are the most relevant rules for understanding the historical development of the concept of hysteria?

I shall try to show that two classes of rules are especially significant in the formation of behaviour which has been variously labelled 'witchcraft', 'hysteria', and 'mental illness'. One pertains to the helplessness of the child and to the corresponding, more-or-less biologically required, help-giving activity of the parent. This results, especially among human beings, in complicated patterns of paired activities *characterized by the helplessness of one member and the helpfulness of the other*.

The second source of rules pertinent to this problem are the teachings and practices of the Judaeo-Christian religions. For centuries Western man has been immersed in an ocean of unserviceable social rules in which he has had to struggle to keep afloat and has nearly drowned. What I mean by this is that, through the combined impact of ubiquitous childhood experiences of dependence and of religious teachings, social life is so structured that it contains endless exhortations commanding man to behave childishly, stupidly, and irresponsibly. These exhortations to helplessness, although perhaps more powerful in their impact during former historical periods, have continued to influence human behaviour to the present day.

I will illustrate the thesis that we are afloat in a vast but unperceived ocean of human commands to be incompetent, impoverished, and sick mainly by references to the New Testament. In each person's actual life experiences, however, such influences need not necessarily come from formally organized religious sources. On the contrary, they more often derive from one's father, mother, husband, wife, employer, and so on. However, the roles of the priest and of the physician are especially significant in this connection, since their succouring activities rest squarely on the premise that the sinful, the weak, the sick – in brief, the disabled – should be helped. By implication, those who exhibit effective, self-reliant behaviour need not be helped. They may even be taxed, burdened, or coerced in various ways. This *rewarding of disability* – however necessary it may sometimes be – is a social practice fraught with complex, unanticipated, and often undesirable consequences.

The Game-playing Model of Behaviour

The communicational frame of reference implies that the communicants are engaged in an activity that is meaningful to them.

By 'meaningful' I refer to purposeful, goal-directed activity, and to the pursuit of goals in certain predetermined ways. If it appears that human beings are not so engaged, it is useful nevertheless to assume that they are, and that we have been unable to comprehend the goals and the rules of their game. This perspective on human behaviour is not novel. Shakespeare said there was 'method in madness'. Similarly, in everyday life when a person acts in an incomprehensible and seemingly senseless fashion, someone might ask: What is his game? or What is his racket? The basic psychoanalytic attitude towards 'neurotic behaviour' reflects the same premise. The analyst tries to understand conduct in terms of unconscious motives, goals, roles, and the like. In the terms proposed here, the analyst seeks to unravel the game of life that the patient plays.

A systematic exposition of the game-playing model of human behaviour, based largely on the works of Mead and Piaget, will form the introduction to this subject. This will be supplemented by the construction of a game-hierarchy, with first-level or *object games* distinguished from higher-level or *metagames*.

Hysteria may be regarded as a heterogeneous mixture of metagames. As such, it – and mental illness generally – may be contrasted with uncomplicated cases of bodily illness and its treatment. The latter, being concerned with bodily survival, may be regarded as an object game.

Attempts simultaneously to pursue object games and metagames may bring a person into irreconcilable conflicts. Patrick Henry's famous declaration, 'Give me liberty or give me death!' illustrates the potential conflict between physical survival and the ethical ideal of liberty. In this example, the end-goal of the metagame – that is, to live as a free man – takes precedence over the end-goal of the object game – that is, to survive at any cost. Conversely, adherence to the subject game in this dilemma implies scuttling the metagame.

Games on any logical level may be played well or poorly. This holds true for hysteria, too. However, inasmuch as hysteria is composed of a mixture of several games, and inasmuch as the person trying to play this complex game is not fully aware of the rules by which he plays and the goals which he has set for himself, there is great likelihood of serious conflict in pursuing the goals and obeying the rules of the several games. This type of analysis will help us to see that while so-called psychiatric problems have significant intrapersonal, interpersonal, and social dimensions, they invariably have ethical dimensions as well. Once man rises above the level of playing the simplest sort of object game – the survival game – he is inevitably confronted by moral choices. Yet the scrutiny of the historical antecedents of 'neurotic symptoms' or 'character' cannot alone resolve an ethical dilemma. This can be accomplished only by making a human choice and committing one's self to it. This does not negate – on the contrary, it re-emphasizes – that the ability and the desire to make choices are themselves influenced by personal experiences.

The game-analytic description of human behaviour unites elements of the sign-using and rule-following models into a coherent whole. This approach to psychiatry is, I believe, especially fitting and useful for an integration of economic, moral, and sociopolitical considerations with the more traditional concerns of the psychiatrist.

BOOK ONE
The Myth of Mental Illness

PART I
Growth and Structure of the Myth

1 Charcot and the Problem of Hysteria

To do justice to the problem of hysteria, the connections between it and malingering must be fully explored. This task requires that we address ourselves to the historical background of this problem. I shall start with the work of Charcot, with whose contributions modern psychiatry can be said to begin, and shall thence trace the development of this theme to the present day.

Charcot on Hysteria

Charcot was a *neurologist*. This meant that his social role was that of a physician specializing in diseases of the nervous system. But what exactly did this mean in his day? Today, when all of medicine is sharply focused on therapy, it is difficult for most of us to picture the situation as I believe it existed then. In Charcot's day neurologists possessed practically no therapeutic methods with which they could appreciably help their patients. Their function, accordingly, was not primarily therapeutic at all. For a man like Charcot, a professor of pathological anatomy at the Sorbonne, his principal responsibilities were scientific and educational. In addition, as a physician in charge of patients at the Salpêtrière, he was involved in the 'care' of patients. While this task had all the appearance of a therapeutic role, it was not really therapeutic in the contemporary sense of this word. Most patients, and particularly those with organic neurological illnesses, were hospitalized chiefly to segregate them from the more normal members of society. Thus, Charcot's (non-private) patients – like the involuntarily hospitalized mental patients today – were segregated not so much because they were ill as because they disturbed others and were too poor and socially unimportant to be cared for by their families or in private institutions.[1] The patients thus came from and were members of a social class much beneath that of the physicians who worked there. What was Charcot's attitude towards his patients? Freud (1893a) answered this question in his obituary of his great teacher:

Having at his disposal a considerable number of patients afflicted with chronic nervous disease he was enabled to take full advantage of his peculiar talent. He was not much given to cogitation, was not of the reflective type, but he had an artistically gifted temperament – as he said himself, he was a '*visuel*', a seer. He himself told us the following about his method of working. He was accustomed to look again and again at things that were incomprehensible to him, to deepen his impression of them day by day until suddenly understanding of them dawned on him. Before his mind's eye, order then came into the chaos apparently presented by the constant repetition of the same symptoms; the new clinical pictures which were characterized by the constant combination of certain syndromes took shape; the complete and extreme cases, the 'types', were then distinguishable with the aid of a specific kind of schematic arrangement, and with these as a starting point the eye could follow down the long line of the less significant cases, the '*formes frustes*', showing some one or other peculiar feature of the type and fading into the indefinite. He called this kind of mental work, in which he had no equal, 'practising nosography' and he was proud of it. (pp. 10–11)

And further on he added:

But to his pupils, who made the rounds with him through the wards of the Salpêtrière – the museum of clinical facts for the greater part named and defined by him – he seemed a very Cuvier, as we see him in the statue in front of the Jardin des Plantes, surrounded by the various types of animal life which he had understood and described; or else he reminded them of the myth of Adam, who must have experienced in its most perfect form that intellectual delight so highly praised by Charcot, when the Lord led before him the creatures of Paradise to be named and grouped. (p. 11)

[1] I have discussed elsewhere (Szasz, 1957d, 1958b) what determines whether a person is considered 'mentally ill' or 'committable', and have emphasized the significance of *power* and *value* in this regard. Thus, today people are segregated in mental hospitals not only because they are 'sick' but also because they are socially unconstructive. This lack of positive contribution to social welfare (however it may be defined) may come about either by default – through stupidity, ineptitude, or lack of human resources – or by rebellion, through the espousal of values and goals too sharply at variance with those dominant in the culture at a given time.

This is an utterly dehumanized view of patients. But then, in some branches of medicine even today, especially in large charity hospitals, patients often are regarded as so much 'clinical material', an expression that clearly betrays the nature of the observer's attitude towards the subject.

I did not, however, cite Charcot's attitude only to criticize it. As will be apparent, these observations are important for an historical analysis of the relationship between malingering and hysteria. For it is clear that if Charcot's principal interest was to classify neurological diseases, he had to scrutinize and distinguish all things that looked like diseases of the nervous system, including those that were, in fact, something else. As the geologist must differentiate gold from copper, and both from other metals which glitter, so the neurologist-nosographer must differentiate multiple sclerosis, tabes, and hysteria. How can he do this?

In Charcot's days the most important tool, besides the clinical examination, was the post-mortem study of the brain. Freud (1893a) provided us with an interesting glimpse of how Charcot carried out his taxonomic work:

During his student days chance brought him into contact with a charwoman who suffered from a peculiar form of tremor and could not get work because of her awkwardness. Charcot recognized her condition to be 'choreiform paralysis', already described by Duchenne, of the origin of which, however, nothing was known. In spite of her costing him a small fortune in broken plates and platters, Charcot kept her for years in his service and, when at last she died, could prove in the autopsy that 'choreiform paralysis' was the clinical expression of multiple cerebro-spinal sclerosis. (pp. 12–13)

Guillain's (1959) biography of Charcot furnishes considerable additional information consistent with the picture sketched so far. For example, we learn that Charcot moved in the highest social circles. He was a friend of Premier Gambetta and also of the Grand Duke Nicholas of Russia. He is said to have paved the way for the Franco-Russian Alliance. By all accounts, he aspired to the role of aristocratic autocrat. It requires no great feat of the imagination to infer what sort of *personal relationship* must have prevailed between him and his destitute and near-illiterate patients.

A firsthand account, although perhaps somewhat embellished, of the human side of Charcot's work may be obtained from Axel

Munthe's beautiful autobiography, *The Story of San Michele* (1930). Of particular interest is Munthe's story of a young peasant girl who took refuge in hysterical symptoms to escape the drudgery of her home life. Munthe felt the 'treatment' she was receiving at the Salpêtrière was making her a lifelong invalid, and that Charcot was, in a way, keeping her imprisoned. He tried to 'rescue' the girl, took her to his apartment, and hoped to convince her to return home. It appears from Munthe's story, however, that the young woman preferred the social role of hysterical patient at the Salpêtrière to that of peasant girl in her village. Evidently, life in the hospital was more exciting and rewarding than her 'normal' existence – a contingency Munthe seriously underestimated. What emerges from this account, too, is that the Salpêtrière, under Charcot, was a special type of social institution. In addition to its similarities to present-day state mental hospitals, its function could also be compared to armies and religious organizations. In other words, the Salpêtrière provided its inmates with certain comforts and gratifications lacking in their ordinary social environment. Charcot and the other physicians who worked there functioned as rulers vis-à-vis their subjects. Instead of intimacy and trust, their relationship to each other was based on fear, awe, and deception.

As Charcot's knowledge of neuropathology increased and as his prestige grew, his interest shifted from neurological disorders to disorders which *simulated* such conditions. Such patients were then classified either hysterics or malingerers, depending on the observer's point of view. Those labelled 'hysterics' were declared relatively more respectable and fit objects for serious study. They were regarded as suffering from an illness, rather than as trying to fool the physician or exhibiting wilful misbehaviour. This is the most fundamental connection, although by no means the only one, between the notions of hysteria and malingering. Freud's account (1893a) of Charcot's work is again illuminating:

He [i.e., Charcot] explained that the theory of *organic nervous diseases* was for the present fairly complete, and he began to turn his attention almost exclusively to *hysteria*, thus suddenly focusing general attention to this subject. This most enigmatic of all nervous diseases – no workable point of view having yet been found from which physicians could regard it – had just at this time come very much into discredit, and this ill-repute related not only to the patients but was extended to the physicians who treated this neurosis. The general opinion was that anything may happen in hysteria; hysterics found no credit whatsoever. *First of all Charcot's work restored dignity to the subject*; gradually the sneering attitude, which the hysteric could reckon on meeting when she told her story, was given up, *she was no longer a malingerer, since Charcot had thrown the whole weight of his authority on the side of the reality and objectivity of hysterical phenomena*. ([Italics added] pp. 18–19)

This passage reveals how the study of hysteria was prejudged because of the importance of its investigator, Charcot. Certain crucial issues were, therefore, obscured and must now be re-examined. Even the simple statement that Charcot turned his attention *to hysteria* rests on the tacit assumption that *this* was the patient's trouble. It was decided by *fiat* that, in contrast to organic neurological diseases, these people had 'functional nervous illnesses'. And most of these 'illnesses' were then named 'hysteria'. Freud's interesting comment should now be recalled: 'hysterics' were no longer diagnosed as malingerers because of Charcot's authority. Freud offered no empirical evidence or logical reason for preferring the category of hysteria to that of malingering. Instead, he appealed to ethical considerations, although without explicitly saying so:

Charcot had repeated on a small scale the act of liberation commemorated in the picture of Pinel which adorned the lecture hall of the Salpêtrière. Now that the blind fear of being fooled by the poor patient which had stood in the way of a serious study of the neurosis was overcome, the question arose which mode of procedure would most speedily lead to the solution of the problem. (p. 19)

This situation is historically significant on two counts: firstly, it marks the beginning of the modern study of so-called mental illnesses; secondly, it contains what I regard as the *major logical and procedural error in the evolution of modern psychiatry*.

Is Every Form of Suffering Illness?

Freud compared Charcot's work to Pinel's. But, as I see it, Pinel's liberation of the mental patient from the dungeon was not a psychiatric achievement at all. It was a moral achievement. He claimed that the sufferers who had been placed in his charge were human beings, and as such entitled to the rights and dignities which, in principle at least, motivated the French Revolution. Pinel did not advocate that the patient should be better treated *because* he was sick. Indeed, the social role of the sick person was not an enviable one at that time. Hence, an appeal for better treatment on this ground would not have been effective.

Pinel's liberation of the mental patient should thus be viewed as social reform rather than as innovation in medical treatment. This is an important distinction. For instance, during the Second World War the removal of venereal infection from the classification of disciplinary offences among military personnel was an act of *social reform*. The discovery of penicillin, while bearing on the same problem – namely, the control of venereal disease – was a *scientific discovery*.

What were the effects of Charcot's insistence that hysterics were ill and not malingering? Although this diagnosis did not alter the hysteric's disability, it did make it easier for him to be 'ill'. Like a little knowledge, this type of assistance can be dangerous. It makes it easier for both sufferer and helper to stabilize the situation and rest content with what is still a very unsatisfactory state of affairs. A comparison of Charcot with another famous French physician, Guillotin, may be illuminating in this connection.

Guillotin's highly questionable contribution to human culture consisted of the reinvention and advocacy of the guillotine. This resulted in a relatively painless and, therefore, less cruel form of execution than those previously in vogue. In our day, the guillotine and the rope have been succeeded in America by the gas chamber and electric chair. Clearly, Guillotin's work is humane or inhuman, depending on which side of the issue we examine. From the point of view of making execution less painful for the executed, it was humane. Since it also made things easier for the executioner and his employers, it was inhuman. What Charcot did was similar. To put it succinctly, *Guillotin made it easier for the condemned to die, and Charcot made it easier for the sufferer, then commonly called a malingerer, to be sick*. It may be argued that when dealing with the hopeless and the helpless, these are real accomplishments. Still, I would maintain that Guillotin's and Charcot's interventions were not acts of liberation, but were rather processes of narcotization or tranquillization.

In short, Charcot and Guillotin made it easier for people – particularly for the socially downtrodden – to be ill and to die. Neither made it easier for people to be well and to live. They used their medical knowledge and prestige to help society shape itself into an image it found pleasing. Efficient and painless execution fitted well into the self-concept of Guillotin's society. Similarly, late nineteenth-century European society was ready to view almost any disability – and particularly one, such as hysteria, that looked so much like a disorder of the body – as illness. Charcot, Kraepelin, Breuer, Freud, and many others lent their authority to the propagation of this socially self-enhancing image of what was then 'hysteria', and what in our day has become the problem of 'mental illness'. The weight of authority of contemporary medical and psychiatric opinion continues, of course, to support and to expand this image.

The practical consequences of the events described are far-reaching for us today. As easy methods of execution have *not* led to the abolition of the death penalty but on the contrary have probably delayed social reforms in this regard, so, I believe, labelling people disabled by problems in living as 'mentally ill' has only impeded and delayed recognition of the essential nature of the phenomena. At first glance, to advocate that an unhappy or troubled person is 'sick' seems 'humane', for it bestows upon him the dignity of suffering from a 'real illness'. But a hidden weight is attached to this viewpoint which pulls the suffering person back into the same sort of disrepute from which this semantic and social reclassification was intended to rescue him.

Another error in decreeing that some malingerers be called hysterics was that it led to obscuring the similarities and differences between organic neurological disease and phenomena that only resembled them. In analysing hysteria, we have a choice between emphasizing the similarities or the differences between it and neurological illness. Actually, both are readily apparent. The *similarities* between hysteria and bodily illness lie chiefly in the patient's complaints, his clinical appearance, and the fact that he is, in fact, disabled. The *differences* between them lie in the empirical findings on physical, laboratory, and post-mortem examination. Moreover, these similarities and differences do not really stand in opposition to one another: there is no reason to believe that every person who complains of being ill or who looks ill or who is disabled – or who manifests all three of these features – must *also* have a physicochemical disorder of his body! This does not deny the possibility that there may be a connection between such complaints and bodily diseases. The nature of this connection, however, is *empirical, not logical*. Once this is clear, it becomes a matter of scientific and social choice whether we prefer to emphasize the similarities – and place hysteria in the category of illness; or whether we prefer to emphasize the differences – and place it in the category of non-illness.

The Double Standard in Psychiatry

The aim of my analysis of the problem of hysteria up to here has been to make explicit the *values* which influenced members of the psychiatric profession in the late nineteenth century. I dwelled on Charcot's attitude towards patients to show, firstly, that he never considered himself to be the patient's agent, and secondly, that his principal goal was to identify accurately specific diseases. As a result, Charcot tended to *define* all of the phenomena he studied as neurological disorders. If this accomplished nothing else, it at least *justified* the attention he paid to these phenomena and the pronouncements he made about them. In this respect, Charcot and his group stood in the same sort of relationship to hysteria as the contemporary physicist stands to nuclear war. The fact that atomic energy is used in warfare does not make international conflicts problems in physics; likewise, the fact that the brain is used in human behaviour does not make moral and personal conflicts problems in medicine.

The point is that the prestige of the scientist – whether of a Charcot or of an Einstein – can be used to lend power to its possessor. He then may be able to achieve social goals that he could not otherwise obtain. Once a scientist becomes so engaged, however, he has a powerful incentive to claim that his opinions and recommendations rest on the same grounds as his reputation! In Charcot's case, this meant that he had to base his case about hysteria on the premise that it was an organic neurological illness. Otherwise, if hysteria and hypnosis were problems in human relations and psychology, why should anyone have taken Charcot's opinions as authoritative? He had no special qualifications or competence in these areas. Hence, had he openly acknowledged that he was speaking about such non-medical matters, he might have encountered serious opposition.

These historical developments lie at the root of a double standard in psychiatry that still persists. I refer to the dual orientation of physicians and psychiatrists to certain occurrences which they encounter in their practices. Charcot's informal, 'off-the record' comment about hysteria illustrates this phenomenon:

Some years later, at one of Charcot's evening receptions, I happened to be standing near the great teacher at a moment when he appeared to be telling Brouardel some very interesting story from his day's work. I hardly heard the beginning, but gradually my attention was seized by what he was saying. A young married couple from the Far East: the woman a confirmed invalid: the man either impotent or exceedingly awkward. '*Tachez donc*,' I heard Charcot repeating, '*je vous assure, vous y arriverez*.' Brouardel, who spoke less loudly, must have expressed his astonishment that symptoms such as the wife's could have been produced in such circumstances. For Charcot suddenly broke in with great animation, '*Mais, dans des cas pareils c'est toujours la chose genitale, toujours ... toujours*'; and he crossed his arms over his stomach, hugging himself and jumping up and down on his toes several times in his own characteristic lively way. I know that for one second I was almost paralysed with amazement and said to myself, 'Well, but if he knows that, why does he never say so?' But the impression was soon forgotten; brain anatomy and the experimental induction of hysterical paralyses absorbed all available interest. (Freud, 1893a, p. 295)

Why was Charcot so insistent? With whom was he arguing? With himself! Charcot must have known that he was deceiving himself when he believed that hysteria was a disease of the nervous system. Herein lies the double standard. The organic viewpoint is dictated by social expediency in so far as the rules of the game of medicine are defined so that adherence to this position will be rewarded.[2] Adherence to the psychological viewpoint is required by the physician's loyalty to the 'truth' and his identification or empathy with the patient. This dichotomy is reflected in the two basic contemporary psychiatric methods, namely, the physicochemical and the psychosocial. In the days of Charcot and Freud, however, only the former was recognized as belonging to science and medicine. Interest in the latter was synonymous with charlatanry and quackery.

Although the problem of malingering will be examined in detail in the next chapter, it is necessary here to say a few words concerning Charcot's view of the relationship between hysteria and malingering. In one of his lectures he said:

This brings me to say a few words about malingering. It is found in every phase of hysteria and one is surprised at times to admire the ruse, the sagacity, and the unyielding tenacity that especially the women, who are under the influence of a severe neurosis, display in order to deceive ... especially when the victim of the deceit happens to be a physician. (Guillain, 1959, pp. 138–9)

Already, during Charcot's lifetime and at the height of his fame, it was suggested, particularly by Bernheim, that the phenomena of hysteria were due to suggestion. It was also intimated that Charcot's demonstrations of hysteria were faked, a charge that has since been fully substantiated. Clearly, Charcot's cheating, or his willingness to be duped – whichever it was seems impossible to ascertain now – is a delicate subject. It was called 'the slight failing of Charcot' by Pierre Marie. Guillain (1959), more interested in the neurological than in the psychiatric contributions of his hero, minimized Charcot's involvement in and responsibility for faking experiments and demonstrations on hypnotism and hysteria. But he was forced to concede that:

[2] Adherence to the organic or physicochemical viewpoint was, and continues to be, dictated also by the difficulty in many cases of differentiating hysteria from, say, multiple sclerosis or brain tumour (especially in their early stages). Conversely, patients with neurological illnesses may also exhibit socalled hysterical behaviour or may show signs of other types of 'mental illness'. This problem of the so-called differential diagnosis between 'organic' and 'psychological' illness has constituted one of the major stumbling blocks in the way of a systematic theory of personal conduct free of brain-mythological components.

Charcot obviously made a mistake in not checking his experiments . . . *Charcot personally never hypnotized a single patient, never checked his experiments* and, as a result, was not aware of their inadequacies or of the reasons of their eventual errors. ([Italics added] p. 174)

To speak of 'inadequacies' and 'errors' here is to indulge in euphemisms. What Guillain described, and what others have previously intimated, was that Charcot's assistants had coached the patients on how to act the role of the hypnotized or hysterical person. Guillain himself tested this hypothesis with the following results:

In 1899, about six years after Charcot's death, I saw as a young intern at the Salpêtrière the old patients of Charcot who were still hospitalized. Many of the women, who were excellent comedians, when they were offered a slight pecuniary remuneration imitated perfectly the major hysteric crises of former times. (p. 174)

Troubled by these facts, Guillain asked himself how this chicanery could come about and how it could have been perpetuated? All of the physicians, Guillain hastened to assure us, 'possessed high moral integrity' (p. 175). He then suggested the following explanation:

It seems to me impossible that some of them did not question the unlikelihood of certain contingencies. Why did they not put Charcot on his guard? The only explanation that I can think of, with all the reservation that it carries, is that they did not dare alert Charcot, fearing the violent reactions of the master, who was called the 'Caesar of the Salpêtrière'. (pp. 175–6)

We must conclude that Charcot's orientation to the problem of hysteria was neither organic nor psychological. He recognized and clearly stated that problems in human relationships may be expressed in hysterical symptoms. The point is that he maintained the medical view in public, for official purposes, as it were, and espoused the psychological view only in private, where such opinions were safe.

The Definition of Hysteria as Illness: a Strategy

My criticism of Charcot rests not so much on his adherence to a conventional medical model of illness for his interpretation of hysteria as on his covert use of scientific prestige to gain certain social ends. What were these ends? They were the acceptance of the phenomena of hypnotism and hysteria by the medical profession in general, and particularly by the French Academy of Sciences. But at what cost was this acceptance won? This question is rarely raised. As a rule, only the conquest over the resistance of the medical profession is celebrated. Zilboorg (1941) described Charcot's victory over the French Academy as follows:

These were the ideas which Charcot presented to Académie des Sciences on February 13, 1882, in a paper on the diverse nervous states determined by the hypnotization of hysterics. One must not forget that the Académie had already condemned all research on animal magnetism three times and that it was a veritable *tour de force* to make the Académie accept a long description of absolutely analogous phenomena. They believed, and Charcot himself believed, that this study was far removed from animal magnetism and was a definite condemnation of it. That is why the Académie did not revolt and why they accepted with interest a study which brought to a conclusion the interminable controversy over magnetism, about which the members of the Académie could not fail to have some remorse. And remorse they well might have, for, from the standpoint of the actual facts observed, Charcot did nothing more than what Georget had asked the Académie to do fifty-six years previously. *Whether one called the phenomenon animal magnetism, mesmerism, or hypnotism, it stood the test of time.* The scientific integrity of the Académie did not. Like a government reluctant, indecisive, and uncertain of itself, it did nothing whenever it was safe to do nothing and yielded only when the pressure of events forced it to act and the change of formulatory cloak secured its face-saving complacency. ([Italics added] pp. 362–3)

I have cited these events in detail because I believe that this 'change of formulatory cloak', which secured the admittance of hysteria into the French Academy, constitutes an historical paradigm. Like the influence of an early but significant parental attitude on the life of the individual, it continues to exert a malignant effect on the later development of psychiatry.

Such 'pathogenic' historical events may be counteracted in one of two ways. The first is by reaction-formation. This means an overcompensation against the original influence. Thus, to correct the early organic bias the significance of psychogenic factors in so-called mental illness is exaggerated. Enormous efforts have been expended in modern psychiatry, psychoanalysis, and psychosomatic medicine to create the impression that 'mental illness is like any other illness'.

The second way to remedy such a 'trauma' is exemplified by the psychoanalytic method itself: by helping the person become explicitly aware of the events that influenced his life in the past, the persistent effects of these events on his future can be mitigated and indeed radically modified. In my epistemological analysis of the problem of mental illness, I have relied in part on the same sort of method and premise – namely, that becoming explicitly aware of the historical origins and philosophical foundations of current psychiatric ideas and practices, we may be in a better position to modify them, if modification is needed, than we would be without such self-scrutiny.

2 Illness and Counterfeit Illness

The Logic of Classification

Von Domarus (1944) interpreted schizophrenic 'thought disorder' as a result of the patient's following non-Aristotelian logic. For example, a schizophrenic may equate a stag with an Indian by focusing on a characteristic common feature – namely, swiftness of movement. On this basis, he classifies both stags and Indians as belonging in the same group.

Aristotelian logic, or what is often loosely called 'normal' or 'adult' logic, consists of deductive reasoning of the following sort. From the major premise that 'All men are mortal' and the minor premise that 'Socrates is a man', we conclude that 'Socrates is mortal'. This logical process presupposes an understanding that the class called 'man' consists of specific individuals, bearing proper names.

It will be shown later (in Part II) that the more primitive type of logical operation, mentioned first, is intimately connected with a simple type of symbolization, namely, that resting on a similarity between the object and the sign used to represent it. Such signs are called *iconic*, because they stand for the object represented much as a photograph stands for the person photographed. Languages composed of iconic signs lend themselves to and are suited mainly for classification on the basis of *manifest* (e.g. structural) *similarities*. On the other hand, logically more complex languages, for example those using conventional signs (words), permit classifying diverse objects and phenomena on the basis of more *hidden* (e.g. functional) *similarities*.

Complex language systems, for example those composed of words or mathematical symbols, lend themselves to the formation of increasingly higher levels of abstraction. Illustrative is the formation of classes, and of classes-of-classes, and so on, in such a way that each higher class contains all the previous classes as members of itself. Thus, John Doe is a member of the class (called 'family') *Doe*. Since all the Does are natives of Vermont, they may be further said to be members of the class *Vermonters*. The next superordinate class could be *Americans*, and the next higher still, *human beings*.

All this is to introduce a logical analysis of the relationship between the notions of malingering, hysteria, and illness. Clearly, the question of whether we classify a bit of behaviour that *looks like* a neurological disorder but is not as 'illness', or as something else, has important implications for the science of human behaviour.

On the Notions of 'Real' and 'False'

Identification and classification are fundamental to the need to order the world about us. This activity of ordering, while of special importance to science, is ubiquitous. For instance, we say that some substances are solid, and others liquid; or, we call certain objects 'money', others 'masterpieces of art', and still others 'precious stones'. Expressed logically, we declare that some things are to be grouped in class A, and others in class non-A. In certain instances it may be difficult to decide if a given item belongs in class A or non-A. This derives from two basic sources. Firstly, in the case of naturally occurring items – for instance, copper and gold – the observer may not possess the knowledge, skill, or tools required to distinguish the two. He may then make the mistake of placing item non-A (copper) in class A (gold).

The second source of difficulty in the work of classification derives from man's intelligent, goal-directed participation in the events that shape his life. Thus, not only can two or more naturally occurring objects or events be similar and present a problem in differentiation, but it is also possible for man deliberately to imitate item X, making it look, as much as possible, like item Y. Everyday language takes cognizance of this. Many words designate a particular kind of relationship between two items, A and B, so that A stands for the specially designated object or event, and B signifies what may be termed 'counterfeit-A'. The latter is characterized by looking, more or less, like A, *this similarity in appearance being deliberately created by a human operator* for some purpose. For example, money may be 'real' or 'counterfeit'; a painting or sculpture may be an 'original' or a 'forgery'; a person may be telling the 'truth' or 'lying'; an individual complaining of bodily symptoms may be a 'sick patient' or a 'healthy malingerer'.

What is the relevance of this discussion of the logic of classification to hysteria and the problem of mental illness? The answer is that if we are to have a clear and meaningful concept of illness as a class of phenomena (say, class A), then we must recognize, firstly, that there are occurrences which look like illness but which may turn out to be something else (class B); and secondly, that there are occurrences which may properly belong in the class of counterfeit illness (class C). All this is logically inherent in classifying certain forms of behaviour as illnesses.

Illness, Counterfeit Illness, and the Physician's Role

Confronted with counterfeit, the observer may be deceived because the imitation is very good, because he is relatively unskilled in differentiating A from non-A, or because he wants to believe that non-A is A. Translating this into the language of bodily versus mental illness, we may assert that the physician may be deceived because certain hysterical or hypochondriacal bodily symptoms might be exceedingly difficult to distinguish from physicochemical disorders; or he may be unskilled in recognizing the manifestations of problems in living and might mistake bodily symptoms for physical illness; or lastly, committed to the role of expert engineer of the body as a physicochemical machine, the physician may believe that all the human suffering he encounters is illness.

On the other hand, the observer may be able to distinguish A from counterfeit-A. Or he may believe that he has distinguished between them when in fact he has not.

The differentiation of A from non-A rests on empirical *observations*, and ends in the rendering of a *judgement*. The observer's role is similar to that of umpire, judge, or expert. For example, a painting may be brought to an art expert, so that he can decide if it is a Renaissance masterpiece or a forgery. He may correctly identify the painting as falling into one or the other category. Or he may err either way. Or he may decide that he cannot determine whether the painting is an original or a forgery. In medical terms, this corresponds to the well-known 'differential diagnosis' between organic and mental disease (including the physician's judgement that he does not know what ails the patient). In this role, the physician functions as expert arbiter. If he limits himself to this role, he will simply classify the item brought to him as either A or non-A (including counterfeit-A) – in other words, the physician will limit himself to telling the patient that the allegedly or apparently diseased body which he has brought for examination is sick or not sick (Szasz, 1956b, 1958c).

If the observer has distinguished – or thinks he has – two classes of items, so that he can identify some as members of class A and others as their imitations, he will usually have certain reactions to his own judgement. His judgement may then be implemented by actions taken towards the items or persons concerned. For example, if money is identified as counterfeit, the police will attempt to arrest the counterfeiters. *What will the physician do when confronted with counterfeit bodily illness?* The physician's behaviour in this situation has varied through the ages. Even today, it depends greatly on the personalities and social circumstances of both doctor and patient. I shall comment only on those reactions to this challenge which are pertinent to our present concerns.

1. The physician may react like the police confronted by a counterfeiter. This was the usual response before Charcot, when hysteria was regarded as the patient's attempt to deceive the doctors. It was as if the patient had been a counterfeiter who wanted to pass his worthless bills to the physician. Accordingly, the doctor's reaction was anger and a desire to retaliate. For real money – that is, real illness – physicians rewarded people. For fake money – that is, fake illness – they punished them. Many physicians still conduct themselves according to these unwritten rules of the Original Medical Game.

2. A pawnbroker, wishing to avoid loaning money on paste jewellery, behaves as if he assumed that all his customers want to defraud him. He considers it his responsibility to protect himself against this hazard. Similarly, the physician confronted by the

hysterical patient may decide that he does not wish to treat him. He sends him away. Such a physician says, in effect: 'I deal only with [real] bodily illness.' He may or may not be aware that, among the problems with which he must deal, there are certain occurrences that look like illnesses but are not.

3. Last, but most important, is the step I believe Charcot took and Freud implemented – a step which complements the rules of the Original Medical Game. In that situation the physician felt as if he had been deliberately defrauded by the patient. To feel that he has not been, he redefines the situation by *changing the rules of the game*. The patient and his behaviour are reclassified, in a fashion that might be paraphrased as follows: 'Under the old rules, illness was considered a physicochemical disorder of the body which manifested itself, or was about to manifest itself, in the form of disability. When disabled, the patient was to be rewarded in certain ways (e.g. he was exempt from working, could expect special protections, etc.). But when he merely imitated being disabled, he was to be considered a malingerer and was to be punished. Under the new rules, however, persons disabled by phenomena which only look like illnesses of the body (i.e. hysteria) will also be classified as ill – that is, as mentally ill – and they will be treated by the same rules that apply to persons who are bodily ill.'

I maintain that Freud did not 'discover' that hysteria was a mental illness. He merely asserted and advocated that so-called hysterics be declared 'ill'. The adjectives 'mental', 'emotional', and 'neurotic' are semantic strategies to codify – and, at the same time, to conceal – the differences between two classes of disabilities or 'problems' in meeting life: one consists of bodily diseases which, by impairing the functioning of the human body as a machine, create difficulties in social adaptation; the other consists of difficulties in social adaptation not attributable to a malfunctioning machinery but 'caused' rather by the purposes the machine was made to serve by those who 'built' it (e.g. parents, society), or by those who 'use' it (i.e. individuals).

To illustrate the far-reaching implications of the foregoing process of reclassification, let us return to our earlier example of the art expert as someone whose job resembles the physician's. The expert may be commissioned to determine whether, for example, a beautiful French painting of uncertain origin was painted by Cézanne, as claimed by the art dealer, or whether it is a forgery, as feared by the prospective buyer. If the expert plays the game properly, he can reach only one of two answers: he concludes either that the painting is a genuine Cézanne 'masterpiece' or that it is a 'forgery'.

But suppose that in the process of examining the painting, studying its origin, and so on, the art expert becomes increasingly impressed by the craftsmanship of the artist, irrespective of who he was, and by the loveliness of his work. Might he not conclude that, although the painting is not a genuine Cézanne, it is nevertheless a 'real masterpiece'? In fact, if the painting is truly excellent, he might even declare that it is a greater masterpiece than a real Cézanne. The artist – let us call him Zeno, hitherto an unknown painter of Greek descent – may then be 'discovered' as a 'great impressionist painter'. But did the expert 'discover' Zeno and his masterpiece? Or did he 'make' him a famous artist, and his painting a valuable canvas, by the weight of his expert opinion, seconded of course by the weight of many other art experts?

This analogy is intended to show that, strictly speaking, no one discovers or makes a masterpiece. And no one 'falls ill with hysteria'. Artists paint pictures, and people become, or act, disabled. But the *names*, and hence the *values*, we give to paintings – and to disabilities – depend on the rules of the system of classification that we use. Such rules, however, are not God-given, nor do they occur 'naturally'. Since all systems of classification are made by people, it is necessary to be aware of who has made the rules and for what purpose. If we fail to take this precaution, we run the risk of remaining unaware of the precise rules we follow, or worse, of mistaking the product of a strategic classification for a 'naturally occurring' event. I believe this is exactly what happened in psychiatry during the past sixty or seventy years during which a vast number of occurrences were reclassified as 'illnesses'. We have thus come to regard phobias, delinquencies, divorce, homicide, addiction, and so on, almost without limit, as psychiatric illnesses. This is a colossal and costly mistake.

But immediately someone might object that this is not a mistake, for does it not benefit addicts, homosexuals, or so-called criminals that they are regarded as 'sick'? To be sure, such relabelling might benefit some people, some times. But this is so largely because people tolerate uncertainty poorly and insist that 'misbehaviour' be classified either as 'sinful' or as 'sick'. This dichotomy must be rejected. Socially deviant or obnoxious behaviour may be classified in numerous ways, or may be left unclassified. Placing some individuals or groups in the class of sick people may indeed be justified by considerations of social expediency but cannot be supported by scientific observations or logical arguments.

For greater precision, we should ask: for whom, or from what point of view, is it a mistake to classify non-illnesses as illnesses? Clearly, it is a mistake from the point of view of science and intellectual integrity. It is also a mistake if we believe that good ends – say, the social rehabilitation of criminals – do not justify the use of morally dubious means; in this case, deliberate, or quasi-deliberate misrepresentation and appeal to false-hood.

This reclassification of non-illnesses as illnesses has, of course, been of special value to physicians and to psychiatry as a profession and social institution. The prestige and power of psychiatrists have been inflated by defining even more phenomena as falling within the purview of their discipline. Thus, Mortimer Adler (1937) has correctly noted that psychoanalysts 'are trying to swallow everything in psychoanalysis' (p. 122). It is difficult to see why we should permit, much less encourage, such expansionism in a profession and a science. In international relations, we no longer treasure the Napoleonic ideal of national expansion at the expense of the integrity of neighbouring peoples. Why, then, do we not consider psychiatric expansion-ism – even though it might be aided and abetted from many

56

sides (by patients, medical organizations, lawyers, etc.) – equally undesirable?

The role of the psychiatric physician as expert arbiter charged with deciding who is or is not ill has not ceased with the renaming of malingering as hysteria and with calling the latter an illness. It has merely made his job more arbitrary and nonsensical.

Let us take a closer look at the logic of reclassifying certain non-illnesses as illnesses. With proper criteria and methods, it is possible to decide that some items are A's, and all others are non-A's. At a later time the basis of our classification may be revised and items from the latter group removed and placed in the former. It must be emphasized that the usefulness of any class and the *name* we give it depends partly on the fact that only a few things are included in it. Of all the colours in the visible spectrum, only a few are called 'green'. If we enlarged the range of colours thus designated, which we could certainly do, we would achieve this at the expense of other colours. It is conceivable, for example, that we should become preoccupied with the similarities between green and other-coloured lights by focusing on the fact that we can see and read by light that is not green also. We may then decide to *call* more and more colours 'green'. If this sort of reasoning were carried to its absurd limits, all colours would be called green. This feat, however, would be accomplished at the cost of obscuring the differences between green and blue, red, violet, etc.

Something of this sort has, in fact, already happened in contemporary medicine and psychiatry. Starting with such things as syphilis, tuberculosis, typhoid fever, and carcinomas and fractures, we have created the class called 'illness'. At first, this class was composed of only a few items, all of which shared the common feature of reference to a state of disordered structure or function of the human body as a physicochemical machine. As time went on, additional items were added to this class. They were not added, however, because they were newly discovered bodily disorders. The physician's attention and interest had been deflected from this criterion and had become focused instead on disability and suffering as new criteria for selection. Thus, at first slowly, such things as hysteria, hypochondriasis, obsessive-compulsive neurosis, and depression were added to the category of illness. Then, with increasing zeal, physicians and especially psychiatrists began to call 'illness' (that is, of course, 'mental illness') anything and everything in which they could detect any sign of 'malfunctioning', based on no matter what norm. Hence, agoraphobia is illness because one should not be afraid of open spaces; homosexuality is illness because heterosexuality is the social norm; divorce is illness because it signals failure of marriage. Crime, art, undesired political leadership, participation in social affairs or withdrawal from such participation – all these things and many more are now said to be symptoms of mental illness.

Three Interpretations of Malingering

Some historical transformations in the concept of malingering illustrate this thesis. The concept of malingering can be shown to reflect the particular ideas which the psychiatrist-as-arbiter holds about what constitutes illness.

Malingering as Simulation of Illness

Before Charcot's time, a person was said to be ill only if his body was physically disordered. Counterfeit illness was called malingering, and the patient so labelled was considered a legitimate object of the physician's scorn. After all, it is our natural reaction to feel anger towards someone who tries to deceive us. Why should physicians behave differently? This, presumably, was the logic that made it acceptable for physicians to act destructively towards such persons. This concept of malingering is so well known that it is unnecessary to document it. It is perhaps less appreciated that this view is still respectable and popular, as the following excerpts from a recent article in the *Journal of the American Medical Association* (Chapman, 1957) illustrate:

Physicians in the United States may be unaware of the patient who spends his time going from place to place, resulting in wide travels, and presenting himself to hospitals, with a fanciful history and extraordinary complaints. It is not uncommon for these patients to have many surgical scars crisscrossing their abdomens, and willingly to allow further surgical procedures to be performed. Regardless of the dangers. Publicizing case histories of such patients seems to be the only way of coping with the problem, which exploits medical services that could be put to better use. (p. 927)

The article concludes with the following paragraph:

The case of a 39-year-old merchant seaman is a remarkable example of hospital vagrancy and spurious hemoptysis. Similar patients in Britain have been said to have Münchausen's syndrome because their wide travels and fanciful histories are reminiscent of the travels and adventures of fiction's Baron Münchausen. Such patients constitute an economic threat and an extreme nuisance to the hospital they choose to visit, for their deception invariably results in numerous diagnostic and therapeutic procedures. Publicizing their histories in journals, thereby alerting the medical profession, seems the only effective way of coping with them. *Appropriate disposition would be confinement in a mental hospital.* Such patients have enough social and *mental quirks to merit permanent custodial care*, otherwise their exploitation of medical facilities will go on indefinitely. ([Italics added] p. 933)

These excerpts also illustrate that physicians often play the medical game without self-reflection, unaware of the rules by which the game is played. Finally, it is interesting to note that the author advocates 'permanent custodial care' [sic] as the proper punishment – although he calls it 'care' – of those persons who try to deceive physicians into believing they are sick. Since physicians often have the social power to make such punishment enforceable, this view is not without serious consequences.

Malingering as Conscious Imitation of Illness

With Freud and psychoanalysis a new system of classification came into being. Bodily illness was class A. Hysteria was still regarded as a form of counterfeit illness, but a very special form of it indeed: the patient himself did not know that he was simulating! Hysteria was thus viewed as *unconscious* malingering. This was class B. The concept of malingering was still retained, but the arbiter was instructed, so to speak, to diagnose this condition only when the imitation was *conscious*. This new version of malingering (class C) differed from the previous notion of counterfeit illness (of the body) by virtue of the new dichotomy 'conscious-unconscious'.

The role of the psychiatrist-arbiter changed accordingly: previously his task was to distinguish bodily illness from all that did not fit into this class; now it became, in addition to this, also the differentiation of 'unconscious imitation of illness' or 'hysteria' from 'conscious imitation of illness' or 'malingering'. The degree of arbitrariness or error to which these new judgements are open is, of course, even greater than was the case previously. This conceptualization and its subsequent developments lent themselves to an increasingly capricious usage of the concepts of hysteria, neurosis, and mental illness. The difficulties inherent in these arbitrary and vague designations and classifications are all around us. For example, Freud (1928) himself asserted that 'There are people who are complete masochists without being neurotic' (p. 224). But he never explained which masochists are neurotic and which are not.

Malingering as Mental Illness

The inclination to regard virtually all forms of human conduct as illness – especially if they are unusual or are studied by the psychiatrist – is reflected by the contemporary psychoanalytic view of malingering. According to it, malingering is an illness – in fact, an illness 'more serious' than hysteria. This is an interesting logical position, for it amounts to nothing less than a complete denial of man's ability to imitate – in this instance, to imitate certain forms of disability. When simulation of mental illness is regarded as itself a form of mental illness, the rules of the psychiatric game are so defined as explicitly to exclude the class of 'counterfeit illness'. Only two classes are recognized: A – illness, and non-A – non-illness. *Counterfeit illness, or malingering, is now a species of illness. The good imitation of a masterpiece is redefined as itself a masterpiece!* Since a good imitation of a master-piece is as pleasing to the eye as the original this is not an entirely unreasonable point of view. But it entails a radical redefinition of the idea of a 'forgery'. In the case of so-called psychiatric illness, such redefinitions apparently occurred without anyone quite realizing what had happened.

It was probably Bleuler (1924) who first suggested that the simulation of insanity be regarded as a manifestation of mental illness. He wrote: 'Those who simulate insanity with some cleverness are nearly all psychopaths and some are actually insane. Demonstration of simulation, therefore, does not at all prove that the patient is mentally sound and responsible for his actions' (p. 191).

The view that malingering is a form of mental illness became popular during the Second World War (especially among American psychiatrists), when it was believed that only a 'crazy' or 'sick' person would malinger. Eissler (1957) offered a vigorous exposition of this view. He wrote:

It can be rightly claimed that *malingering is always the sign of a disease often more severe than a neurotic disorder* because it concerns an arrest of development at an early phase. *It is a disease* which to *diagnose* requires particularly keen *diagnostic acumen.* The *diagnosis* should never be made but by the *psychiatrist.* It is a great mistake to make a patient suffering from the disease liable to *prosecution,* at least if he falls within the type of personality I have described here. ([Italics added] pp. 252–3)

This proposition has obvious advantages, for it buttresses the potentially shaky morale of the erstwhile civilian physician conscripted into the military service. It supports – at the patient's expense, of course – the physician's covert endorsement of the aims and values of the war effort. Although the patient might have been treated more or less kindly when regarded as 'sick', he was at the same time deprived of this particular opportunity to rebel against the demands placed on him. This form of protest was disallowed, and those who resorted to it were demoted and disenfranchised by being labelled 'mentally ill', by being given 'N.P. discharges', and by similar methods of disguised punishment.

Concluding Remarks on Objects and their Representations

The unifying thread that runs through this chapter is the notion of similarity. An iconic sign – say a photograph – resembles the object it represents. So does a map the terrain of which it is a two-dimensional model. It should be recalled that the proper use of a photograph or a map implies that they merely represent real things. In our everyday life, it makes a vast practical difference whether objects are clearly recognized as representations or accepted as real – that is, as objects in their own rights. This may be illustrated by contrasting stage money with counterfeit money. Although stage money might look like real money, it is at the same time clearly identified as make-believe. Sometimes the clarity or ambiguity of this identification might be a matter of controversy. For instance, we could imagine a situation in which stage money was mistaken for real money. The point to be emphasized here is that *the context of a message forms an integral part of the total communicational package*. Thus, whether bills are regarded as stage money or counterfeit may depend not so much on how the objects appear as on who passes them to whom, where, and how. The stage setting itself implies that the monies used are props. Similarly, the setting of an economic transaction implies that the monies are real, and if they are not real, that they are counterfeit.

Let us apply these considerations to the problem of hysteria. Now it is disabled behaviour that is under scrutiny, but the communicational package must include *the situation in which such behaviour is presented*. If it is presented in a physician's office, we must ask: should the disabled behaviour be viewed as an object in its own right, or as a representation? If the phenomena presented are regarded and treated as real objects, then they must be classified as illness or as malingering, depending solely on one's definition of what constitutes illness. If, however, the phenomena are regarded as the representations (models or signs of other occurrences) – then a totally different interpretation becomes possible. We may now speak of illness-imitative behaviour. This, however, can under no circumstances be called illness unless we are prepared to commit the logically nonsensical operation of placing an item and its known imitation in the same class.

Agreeing to the proposition that both malingering and hysteria refer to illness-imitative behaviour, we are still left with some uncertainties concerning the cognitive quality (i.e. the degree of 'consciousness') and the intent of the imitation. In the case of stage money, we know that both actors and spectators are aware that what looks like money is in fact an imitation – a prop. In contrast, the term 'counterfeit' implies that only the counter-feiters know that it is a facsimile, whereas those who receive it, and who then might even pass it on to others, do not know this. They believe that they possess the object proper when they hold merely its imitation. In short, they are deceived.

What is the comparable situation in the case of hysteria? Does the patient believe that he is ill (object proper), or that he is offering a representation (facsimile) of illness? Some insist that the patient offers illness in good faith; others argue that he knows he is not ill. These two divergent answers reflect the difference between the diagnoses of hysteria and malingering. There is evidence to support both of these positions. The question raised cannot, therefore, be answered unequivocally. Indeed, the patient's failure to define his message either as object or as representation constitutes one of the crucial character-istics of his behaviour. (This problem will be examined further in Part IV; see especially Chapter 13.)

So much for the patient, in his role as actor or message-sender. What about the spectators – the recipients of the message? The spectator's reaction to the drama of hysteria will depend on his personality and relationship to the actor (patient). Stranger and relative, foe and friend, non-psychiatric physician and psychoanalyst – each will react differently. I shall comment briefly on the reactions of the last two only. The non-psychiatric physician tends to treat all forms of disability as objects proper, not as representations. That is, he tends to view all forms of disability as illness or potential illness. On the other hand, the psychoanalyst, in his actual work with the patient, will tend to treat all phenomena as representations. But since he has failed to codify clearly this logical distinction, he will persist in de-scribing his observations, and his theories about them, as if he were talking about objects instead of representations. Representa-tions are no less real, of course, than real objects. A photograph of John Doe is just as real as is John Doe in the flesh. But the two are obviously not the same; nor do they belong in the same class.

If we take this distinction between objects and their repre-sentations seriously, we shall be compelled to regard psychiatry as dealing with communications or sign-using behaviour, *not* with mental illness. Accordingly, psychiatry and neurology are not sister sciences, both belonging to the super-ordinate class called medicine. Rather, psychiatry stands in a *meta relation* to neurology and to other branches of medicine. Neurology is concerned with certain parts of the human body and its functions *qua* objects in their own rights – *not* as signs of other objects. Psychiatry (as defined here) is expressly concerned with signs *qua* signs – not merely with signs as things pointing to objects more real and interesting than they themselves.

3 Sociology of the Therapeutic Situation

Traditionally, psychiatrists have regarded mental illness as a problem apart from and independent of the social context in which it occurred. The symptomatic manifestations of diseases of the body, for instance of diphtheria or syphilis, are indeed independent of the sociopolitical conditions of the country in which they occur. A diphtheritic membrane was the same and looked the same whether it occurred in a patient in Tsarist Russia or Victorian England.

Since mental illness was considered to be basically like bodily illness, it was logical that no attention was paid to the social conditions in which the alleged disease occurred. This is not to say that the effects of social conditions on the causation of illness were not appreciated. On the contrary, this sort of relationship had been recognized since antiquity. However, although it was known that poverty and malnutrition favoured the development of tuberculosis, or sexual promiscuity the spread of syphilis, it was nevertheless held that once these diseases made their appearance their *manifestations* were the same whether the patient was rich or poor, nobleman or serf. Although the phenomenological features of bodily illnesses are independent of the socio-economic and political structure of the society in which they occur, this is not true of so-called mental illnesses. The manifestations of psychosocial disabilities vary in accordance with educational, socio-economic, religious, and political factors.

When persons belonging to different religious and socio-economic groups become bodily ill – for example, with pneumonia or bronchogenic carcinoma – their bodies manifest the same sort of physiological derangements. Hence, in principle, for given diseases all patients might receive the same treatments, irrespective of who they are. Indeed, this is the scientifically correct

65

position with respect to physicochemical disturbances of the body. This medical standard of treatment has, however, been applied to so-called mental illnesses, to which, in my opinion, it does not apply. To understand why it does not, it is necessary to examine and make explicit how therapeutic attitudes – or, more precisely, physician–patient relationships – vary in accordance with historical and sociopolitical circumstances. To do this, the characteristic therapeutic situations of three different socio-cultural settings will be briefly described and analysed. They are: (1) late nineteenth-century, Western European medicine; (2) medical practice in contemporary Western democracies, especially in the United States; and (3) Soviet medical practice.

The term 'therapeutic situation' will be used to refer to medical and psychotherapeutic practice. Since the inter-relations of social structure, value, and therapeutic situation are numerous and complex, two clearly identifiable aspects of the general problem will be selected for special attention. They may be stated in the form of questions: (1) Whose agent is the therapist (physician, psychotherapist, etc.)? (2) How many persons, or institutions, are directly involved in the therapeutic situation?

Nineteenth-century Liberalism, Capitalism, and Individualism

Since antiquity, medical care was regarded much as were other economic goods or services. It was a commodity that could be purchased by the rich only. To the poor, when given it had to be given free, as charity. This social arrangement was firmly established by the time modern scientific advances in medicine began, during the latter half of the nineteenth century. It should be recalled, too, that this period was characterized by the rapid flowering of liberal thoughts and deeds in Europe, as manifested, for example, by the abolition of serfdom in Austria-Hungary and Russia.

As industrialization and urbanization flourished, the proletariat replaced the unorganized and sociopsychologically less well-defined peasant class. Thus, a self-conscious and class-conscious capitalism developed, and with it recognition of a new form of mass suffering and disability, namely, poverty. The phenomenon of poverty, as such, was of course nothing new. However, the existence of huge numbers of impoverished people, crowded together within the confines of a city, was new. At the same time, and undoubtedly out of the need to do something about mass poverty, there arose 'therapists' for this new 'disease' of the masses. Among them, Karl Marx is, of course, the best known. He was no solitary phenomenon, however, but rather exemplified a new social role and function – the revolutionary as 'social therapist'. Along with these developments, the ethic of individualism was also strongly bolstered. The basic value of the individual – as opposed to the interests of the masses or the nation – was emphasized, especially by the upper social classes. The professions, medicine foremost among them, espoused the ethical value of individualism. This value gradually became pitted against its antonym, collectivism. Although the ethics of individualism and collectivism are polar opposites, their present forms were achieved through a simultaneous development, and they often exist side by side. This was already the case, to some extent, in the days of Charcot, Breuer, and Freud. This contention may be illustrated by some observations concerning the therapeutic situations characteristic of that period.

The physician in Charcot's Paris, or in his counterpart's Berlin, Moscow, or Vienna, was usually engaged in two diametrically opposite types of therapeutic practices or situations. In one, he was confronted by an affluent private patient. This meant that he served, by and large, as the patient's agent, having been hired by him to make a diagnosis and, if possible, achieve a cure. The physician, in turn, demanded payment for services rendered. He thus had an economic incentive, in addition to other incentives, to help his patient. Furthermore, since some bodily illnesses were considered shameful (including not only venereal diseases but tuberculosis and certain dermatological ailments as well), a wealthy person could also avail himself of the social protection of privacy. As a rich man could buy a house large enough to provide several rooms for his sole occupancy, so also he could buy the services of a physician for his sole use. In its extreme form, this amounted to having a personal physician, much as one had a valet, maid, or cook. This custom is by no means extinct. In some parts of the world, wealthy or socially prominent people still have personal physicians whose duty is to care only for them or perhaps their families.

A similar, but less extreme, arrangement is afforded by the private, two-person medical situation. This arrangement insures for the patient the time, effort, and privacy which he considers necessary for his care and still allows the physician to care for other patients within the limits of his available time and energy. The development of privacy as an integral part of the (private) therapeutic situation seems to be closely tied to the capitalistic economic system. The Hippocratic oath commands the physician to respect and safeguard the patient's confidential communications. The Greek physician of antiquity practised, of course, in a capitalist society, selling his services to the rich, and helping the poor without recompense.

It is implicit in this discussion that having access to a private therapeutic relationship is desirable. Why is this sort of privacy desired? The answer lies in the connections between illness (or disability) and shame, and between shame and privacy. The feeling of shame is closely related to what other people think of one. Exposure and humiliation are feared both as punishments for shameful acts and as stimuli for increasingly intense feelings of shame. Secrecy and privacy protect the person from public exposure and hence from shame. Regardless of whether the shame is occasioned by physical disability, psychological conflict, or moral weakness, it is more easily acknowledged if it is shared with only a single person – as it is in the confessional or in private psychotherapy – than if it is communicated to many people. Privacy in medical or psychotherapeutic relationships is thus useful because it protects the patient from undue embarrassment and humiliation, and thus facilitates psychological mastery of the problem.

In addition, privacy and secrecy in the therapeutic situation are desirable and necessary also to protect the patient from 'real' – that is, social rather than intrapersonal – dangers. Social isolation and ostracism, loss of employment, and injury to family and social status are some of the hazards that threaten a person should his condition or diagnosis become public knowledge. In this connection, such possibilities as syphilis in a schoolteacher, psoriasis in a cook, or schizophrenia in a judge should be kept in mind. These, however, are merely illustrative examples. The possibilities both of reward and penalty for publicly established diagnoses are virtually limitless. The precise character of the rewards and penalties will vary, once again, with the moral, political, and scientific character of the society.

The second type of therapeutic situation I want to consider is charity practice. The differences between it and private practice are often overlooked as a result of concentrating on the patient's disease and the physician's alleged desire to cure it. In traditional charity practice, the physician was not principally the patient's agent. Sometimes he was not the patient's agent at all. Accordingly, a truly confidential relationship between patient and physician could not develop. The physician was technically and legally responsible to his superiors and employers. He was, therefore, bound to orient himself for his rewards, at least to some extent, to his employer, rather than to his patient. It is often maintained nowadays that removing the financial involvement with the patient enables the physician better to concentrate on the technical task at hand (provided that he is adequately remunerated). While this might well be true in thoracic surgery, it is assuredly not true in psychoanalysis. In any case, it is clear that the financial inducement which the private patient offers the physician is absent in charity practice. The main features of these two types of therapeutic situations are summarized in Table 1.

The contrast between private and public medical care is often represented as if it were like the difference between a palace and a hovel. One is fine and expensive; anyone who could afford to secure it would be foolish if he did not do so, especially if he needed it. The other is inferior and second-rate; at best, it makes life livable. Hence, although physicians and politicians have always assured the poor that their medical care was equally as good as that of the rich, more often than not this message fell on deaf ears. Instead of accepting this pious message, people have tried to raise their standard of living. In this effort, so far the people of the United States and some European countries have been most successful. This has resulted in certain fundamental

69

Characteristics of the Situation	*Private Practice*	*Charity Practice*
Number of participants	Two (or few) Two-person situation 'Private'	Many Multiperson situation 'Public'
Whose agent is the therapist?	Patient's Patient's guardian's (e.g. paediatrics) Patient's family's	Employer's (e.g. institution, state, etc.)
Sources and nature of the therapist's rewards	Patient: money, referrals, etc.	Employer: money, promotion, prestige through status
	Patient's relatives and friends: satisfaction from having helped	Patient's relatives and friends: satisfaction from having helped
	Self: satisfaction from mastery	Self: satisfaction from mastery
	Colleagues: satisfaction from proven competence	Colleagues: satisfaction from proven competence

changes in the patterns of medical care – and hence in the sociology of the therapeutic situation – in these countries. I shall comment on these changes now, and shall then consider medical developments in the Soviet Union.

Contemporary Society and Its Patterns of Health Care

Progressive technological and sociocultural sophistication has led to the development of several means of protection against future poverty, want, and helplessness. One of these is insurance. We shall here be especially concerned with the effects of health insurance on medical and psychotherapeutic relationships.

Insured Practice

From our present point of view it matters little whether protection from illness is guaranteed for the individual by a private insurance company or is furnished by the state. Health protection by means of privately purchased insurance is in the tradition of private ownership and capitalism and is, accordingly, popular in the United States. Protection by means of taxation and socialized medicine has been the method chosen in Great Britain. To most Americans, this appears to be more socialistic and hence bad. It is essential to discard these clichés, so that we can address ourselves to the relevant variables in these situations.

Health insurance introduces a completely new phenomenon into the practice of medicine. The most significant feature of insured practice – a name which I suggest to distinguish it from both private and charity practice – is that *it is neither private nor public*. The physician–patient relationship is so structured that the doctor is neither the patient's nor a charitable institution's sole agent. This arrangement cannot be reduced to the old patterns of medical care, nor can it be understood in their terms. It is commonly believed that the insured situation does not differ significantly from the private practice situation, the only difference being that the physician is paid by the insurance company instead of by the patient. Rarely is insured medicine regarded as similar to charity practice. I submit, however, that there are more important similarities between insured and charity practice than between insured and private practice. For the insurance arrangement, like the charitable one, makes a two-person, confidential relationship between doctor and patient virtually impossible.

Without penetrating further into the sociological intricacies of insured medicine, I should like to offer some generalizations which may be useful for our understanding of the problem of mental illness. It appears to be a general rule that the more clear-cut, objective, or socially acceptable a patient's disease is, the more closely insured practice resembles private practice. For example, if a housewife slips on a banana peel in her kitchen and fractures her ankle, her treatment may not be significantly influenced by who pays for it – she, or an insurance company, or the state.

On the other hand, the more an illness deviates from something that *happens* to a person, and the more it is something that the person *does* or *makes happen*, the greater are the differences between the insured situation and the private, two-person situation. For instance, if our patient falls in a factory rather than in her kitchen, she will then not only receive compensation but also be granted a medical excuse to stay away from work. And, if, let us say, she has a young child with whom she would like to spend more time at home, she will have a strong incentive to be disabled for more than a minimum length of time. Obviously, this sort of situation requires an arbiter or judge to decide whether a person is or is not disabled ('sick'). The physician is generally regarded as the proper person for this task. It may be argued that physicians in private practice also play this role. But this is not so. The physician in private practice is primarily the patient's agent. Should there be a conflict between his opinion and the presumed 'real facts' – as may occur when the patient is involved with life insurance companies, draft boards, or industrial concerns – the latter groups rely on the judgements of *their own physicians*. In the case of the draft board, for example, the examining physician has absolute power to overrule a private physician's opinion. And if he does not have such power, as in the case of an industrial concern, the conflict of interests is arbitrated in a court of law.

In the case of insured practice, the answer to the question, Whose agent is the physician? is not clearly defined. As a result, it is possible for the physician to shift from one position to another. He may act entirely on behalf of the patient one minute, and line up against him the next.[1]

As a third generalization, I would state that so-called mental illnesses share only a single significant characteristic with bodily diseases: the sufferer or 'sick person' is more or less disabled from performing certain activities. The two differ in that mental illnesses can be understood only if they are viewed as occurrences that do not merely happen to a person but rather are brought

[1] The terms 'for' or 'against' the patient, and 'good' or 'bad' for him, are used here solely in accordance with the patient's own definition of his wants and needs. Any other definition, such as attempting to determine whether the therapist is acting on behalf of, or opposed to, the patient in accordance with the therapist's avowed intentions, can lead only to confusion and social exploitation. A good example is the notion that all psychiatrists are 'therapists' acting on behalf of the patient's best interests, irrespective of what they in fact do (Szasz, 1957d, 1960d).

about by him (perhaps unconsciously), and hence are of some value to him. This assumption is not necessary – indeed, it is insupportable – in the typical cases of bodily illness.

The premise that the behaviour of persons said to be mentally ill is meaningful and goal-directed – provided one is able to understand the patient's behaviour from *his* particular point of view – underlies all 'rational' psychotherapies. Moreover, if the psychotherapist is to perform his task properly, he must not be influenced by socially distracting considerations concerning his patient. This condition can be met best if the relationship is rigidly restricted to the two people involved in it.

The Private Practice Situation

It is necessary now to refine our conception of private practice. Thus far, this term has been used in its conventional sense to denote the medical activities of any physician *not employed* by an institution or agency (e.g. a company or labour union). According to this definition, such a physician is engaged in private practice, irrespective of how or by whom he is paid. This common-sense definition will no longer suffice. Instead, we shall have to adopt a more limited definition of private practice, based on strict pragmatic criteria. Let us define the Private Practice Situation as *a contract between patient and physician*: the patient hires the doctor to help him with his own health care and pays him for it. If the physician is hired by someone other than the patient, or is paid by another party, the medical relationship will no longer fall in the category of Private Practice Situation. This definition highlights, firstly, *the two-person nature of the relationship*, and secondly, *the autonomy and self-determination of the patient* (Szasz, 1957b, 1959g). I shall continue to use the expression 'private practice' in its conventional sense, to refer to all types of non-charity, non-institutional practice. The term Private Practice Situation (with initials capitalized) will be used to designate the two-person therapeutic situation described above (see Table 2).

It is important to note, in this connection, that affluence fosters not only health insurance but also private practice. In the United States, a considerable proportion of the latter is

Characteristics of the Situation	Private Practice Situation	Insured Practice
Number of participants	Two Two-person situation	Three or more Multiperson situation
Whose agent is the therapist?	Patient's	Therapist's role is poorly defined and ambiguous: Patient's agent, when in agreement with his aspirations Society's agent, when in disagreement with patient's aspirations His own agent, trying to maximize his own gains (e.g. compensation cases)
Sources and nature of therapist's rewards	Patient: money, referrals, etc. Self: satisfaction from mastery Colleagues	Patient: cure, gratitude, etc. Self: satisfaction from mastery Colleagues System or state: money, promotion, etc.

psychiatric or psychotherapeutic practice. This proportion becomes even more significant if it is considered not in relation to the general category of private practice, but rather in relation to the narrowly defined Private Practice Situation. Indeed, I believe that psychotherapeutic practice is the most important contemporary (American) representative of a truly two-person therapeutic relationship. Deterioration in the privacy of the traditional (nineteenth-century) medical situation may have been one of the stimuli for increasing the demand for psychotherapeutic services. Since the general physician ceased to be the true representative of the patient, the suffering person has turned to the psychiatrist and to the nonmedical psychotherapist as new representatives of his best interests.

I do not wish to imply that deterioration in the privacy of the medical situation is largely responsible for the increasing demand for psychotherapeutic help in contemporary America. The role of affluence itself is probably significant in this connection, for as soon as people have more money than they need for the so-called necessities of life (whatever these may be), they will expect to be 'happy'. And they will then use some of their money to seek 'happiness'. The social function of psychotherapy, from this point of view, must be compared not only with that of religion but also with that of alcohol, tobacco, cosmetics, and various recreational activities.

These considerations touch on the relationship between social class, mental illness, and the type of treatment received for it, a subject recently explored by Hollingshead and Redlich (1958). These authors found, for example, that affluent psychiatric patients tend to receive psychotherapy, while poor patients are treated with physical interventions. Psychological help and physical therapies represent so grossly different types of psychiatric interventions that no meaningful comparison about which is 'better' can be made between them. Hollingshead and Redlich's findings demonstrate, however, that there are significant connections between economic status, education, and a self-responsible, self-determinate mode of orienting one's self to a help-seeking situation. I emphasize this because I believe that the social impact of the affluent society on psychiatry (and on medicine, generally) is such as both to foster and inhibit the growth of a two-person therapeutic situation. Better education and economic security favour the conditions necessary for a two-person therapeutic contract. At the same time, the spread of insured health protection, whether through private insurance, veterans' benefits, or government-sponsored medical care, creates a new type of therapeutic relationship that tends to preclude a truly two-person arrangement.

Finally, it is worth noting that while the Private Practice Situation is being displaced by insured patterns of care in the democracies, in the Soviet Union it was displaced when physicians became employees of the state. Medical practice in Soviet Russia will now be examined to contrast the role of the physician as agent of the patient with his role as agent of the state.

Soviet Medicine

The great majority of the Russian population depends on medical services furnished by the state. Private practice exists, but is available only to those occupying the top layers of the Soviet social pyramid. Another crucial feature of the Russian medical scheme is the result of the government's strong emphasis on the production of agricultural, industrial, and other types of goods. The need to work is impressed on the people in every possible way. It follows that for those who wish to avoid working, falling sick and remaining disabled is one of the most important avenues of escape from what they experience as an intolerable demand. Since the presence of sickness is not always obvious to the layman, the physician is chosen as the expert arbiter who must decide which of the persons who claim to be ill are 'really ill', and which ones only 'malinger'. Field (1957) described this as follows:

It stands to reason that certification of illness cannot be left, under most circumstances, to the person who claims to be sick. This would make abuses too easy. It is the physician, then, as the only person technically qualified to do so, who must 'legitimize' or 'certify' sickness in the eyes of society. This means, in turn, that abuses of the patient's role will consist in conveying to the physician the impression that one's sickness is independent of one's conscious motivation – whereas it actually is not. This possibility beclouds the *classical assumption* that the person who comes to the physician must *necessarily* be sick (independently of motivation): on the contrary, in certain cases, just the opposite assumption may be held. This has, of course, important implications for both physician and 'genuine' patient.

It is held here that a society (or social group) which, for any number of reasons, cannot offer its members sufficient incentives of motivation for the faithful and spontaneous performances of their social obligations must rely on coercion to obtain such performances. Because of the presence of coercion such a society will also generate a high incidence of deviant behaviour to escape coercion. *Simulation of illness (technically known as malingering) will be one form of such behaviour. Malingering can be considered as a medical, a social, and a legal problem.* It is a medical problem only insofar as it is the physician's task to certify who is *a bona fide patient* and who is a *faker*. It is a social problem insofar as the assumption that the person who comes to the physician must necessarily be sick (independently of motivation) is no longer tenable. The opposite assumption may sometimes be just as valid. It is often a legal problem because a fraud has been perpetrated.

Malingering may have far-reaching consequences because the 'business' of society (or the group) is not done and because ordinary social sanctions are inadequate to close this escape value. This means, in turn, that some provision must be made, some mechanism devised, to control the granting of medical dispensations. The logical point at which to apply this control is the physician. ([Italics added] pp. 146-8)

According to Field, Russian physicians are afraid to be lenient with patients not demonstrably ill. There is widespread anxiety that every patient is a potential spy or *agent provocateur*.

The social status of the Soviet physician is relatively low. Most of them are women. Their status is similar to that of our social workers or public school teachers. A comparison of American and Soviet medicine raises many questions concerning the merits and shortcomings of public and private systems of education and medical care. I submit that the Soviet physician, the American social worker, and the American public school teacher share a significant common feature: *each functions as an agent of society*. By this I mean that individuals fulfilling these social roles are hired by society or by large social bodies (e.g. a school system), to minister to the needs of group-members (e.g. schoolchildren, persons on relief, the sick, etc.). *They are not hired by their customers, clients, or patients and, accordingly, do not owe their primary loyalties to them.* This arrangement tends to be beneficial to the group as a whole, but is not always advantageous for the specific individuals served. The clash of interests is greatest when the needs of the group and of the individual are widely divergent.

I should now like to call attention to some connections between modern Soviet medicine on the one hand and the social role of the physician in charity practice, say in Charcot's day, on the other hand. The diagnosis of malingering was commonly made in both settings. This was due mainly to two factors: firstly, the physician was an agent of society (or of some part of it), and not of the patient; secondly, the physician tacitly espoused as his own the prevalent social values concerning the patient's productive usefulness in society. The Soviet physician is identified with, and serves the interests of, the communist state; hence he believes, for example, that hard work and productivity are necessary for the welfare of both the individual and society. Similarly, the nineteenth-century, Western physician was identified with, and often served the interests of, the capitalist state; hence he believed, for example, that the woman's 'proper' role was to be wife and mother. Escape from either role – that is, whether from that of downtrodden worker or downtrodden wife and mother – was left open along only a few routes, illness and disability being the chief one.

TABLE 3. SOCIOLOGY OF THE THERAPEUTIC SITUATION
WESTERN VERSUS SOVIET PRACTICE

Characteristics of the Situation	*Western Practice*	*Soviet Practice*
Number of participants	Two or few Private, insured state-supported	Many State-supported
Whose agent is the therapist?	Patient's Employer's His own	Society's Patient's (in so far as patient is positively identified with the values of the state)
	Physician's role is ambiguous	*Physician's role is clearly defined as agent of society*
Ethical basis of therapeutic actions	Individualistic	Collectivistic
Diagnoses encouraged or permitted	Mental illness The sick society	Malingering Psychiatric diagnoses couched in physiologic terms
Diagnoses most avoided or considered non-existent	Malingering	Mental illness (as problem in living)
Relative social status of physician	High	Low

The following quotation from Field (1957) illustrates how strongly the Soviet physician is committed to the role of agent of society, if necessary in opposition to the individualistic needs of any particular patient.

It is perhaps significant to note that the *Hippocratic oath*, which was taken by tsarist doctors (as it is in the West), *was abolished after the revolution because it 'symbolized' bourgeois medicine* and was considered incompatible with the spirit of Soviet medicine. 'If,' continues a Soviet commentator in the *Medical Worker*, 'the prerevolutionary physician was proud of the fact that for him "medicine" and nothing else existed, the Soviet doctor on the other hand is proud of the fact that he actively participated in the building of socialism. *He is a worker of the state*, a servant of the people ... *the patient is not only a person, but a member of socialist society.*' ([Italics added] p. 174)

The Hippocratic oath was abolished, I submit, not because it symbolized 'bourgeois medicine' – for charity practice is as much a part of bourgeois medicine as private practice – but rather because the oath tends to define the physician as an agent of the patient. For the Hippocratic oath is, among other things, a Bill of Rights for the patient. In short, the conflict with which the Russian physician struggles is an ancient one – the conflict between individualism and collectivism. (An abbreviated summary of the constrasting characteristics of Western and Soviet medical systems is presented in Table 3.)

The Significance of Privacy in the Physician–Patient Relationship

Two features of Soviet medicine – firstly, the Russian physician's fear lest by being sympathetic with an *agent-provocateur*-malingerer he bring ruin on himself, and secondly, the abolition of the Hippocratic oath – make it necessary to examine further the role of privacy in the therapeutic situation. The first shows that *the privacy of the physician–patient relationship is not solely for the benefit of the patient*. The belief that it is stems, in part, from the Hippocratic oath, which explicitly asserts that the physician shall not abuse the patient's trusted communications. The contemporary legal definition of confidential communications (to physicians) lends support to this view, since it gives the patient the power to waive confidentiality. Thus, the patient is the 'owner' of his confidential communications. He is in control of when and how this information will be used, or when it shall be withheld.

However, in a psychoanalytic contract – at least as I understand it (Szasz, 1957b, 1959c) – the privacy of the relationship implies that the therapist will not communicate with others, irrespective of whether or not the patient gives permission for the release of information. Indeed, even the patient's pleading for such action on the part of the analyst must remain frustrated, if the two-person character of the relationship is to be preserved.

The common-sense view that confidentiality serves solely the patient's interests makes it easy to overlook the fact that the privacy of the physician–patient relationship provides indispensable protection for the therapist as well. By making the patient a responsible participant in his own treatment, the therapist is protected, to some extent, against the patient's (and the patient's family's, or society's) accusations of wrongdoing. If at all times the patient is kept fully informed as to the nature of the treatment, it will be his responsibility, at least in part, constantly to assess his therapist's performance, to demand changes whenever they appear necessary, and, finally, to leave his therapist should he feel that he is not receiving the help he needs.

There appears to be an inherent conflict between the benefits which the patient may derive from a private, two-person arrangement and the guarantees of protection afforded him by a measure of therapeutic publicity (the latter providing certain official, socially administered checks on the capabilities and performances of the therapist). In a private situation, the patient himself must protect his interests. Should he feel that his therapist has failed him, his chief weapon is to sever the relationship. Likewise, severing the relationship is the only protection for the (psychoanalytic) therapist, for he cannot coerce the patient into 'treatment' by enlisting the help of others, for example, family members. In sharp contrast to the privacy of the psychoanalytic situation, the publicity of the Soviet therapeutic situation fosters the use of mutually coercive influences on the parts of both patient and doctor. Thus, physicians can force patients to do various things by certifying or not certifying their illnesses; while patients, in revenge as it were, are provided with wide latitude for denouncing physicians and bringing charges against them (Field, 1957, pp. 176–7).

These observations also help to account for the non-existence of psychoanalysis, or of any other type of private psychotherapy, in the Soviet Union. The incompatibility of communism and psychoanalysis has been attributed to the communist claim that problems in living are due to the inequities of the capitalist social system. It seems to me, however, that the core of the conflict between psychoanalysis and communism is the privacy of the analytic situation.

Medical Care as a Form of Social Control

It is evident that anything that affects large numbers of people, and over which the state (or the government) has control, may be used as a form of *social control*. In the United States, for example, taxation may be used to encourage or inhibit the consumption of certain goods. Since Russian medical services are operated by the state, they may readily be used for the purpose of contolling individuals and moulding society.

The frequent use of malingering as a medical diagnosis in the Soviet Union suggests that organized medicine is used as, among other things, a form of social tranquillization. In this regard, the similarities between Russian medicine and American social work are especially significant. Both are systems of social care. Both fulfil certain basic human needs, while at the same time both may be used – and, I believe, are used – to exert a subtle but powerful control on those cared for. In Russia, it is the state that employs the physicians, and thus may use them to control the population – for example, by means of a diagnosis of malingering. In the United States, state or local governments or private philanthropic agencies (supported by the upper classes) employ social service workers. This arrangement empowers the employers to exert a measure of social control – in this case, over members of the lower classes. Both systems – that is, Soviet medicine and American social work – are thus admirably suited for the purpose of keeping 'in line' potentially discontented members (or groups) of society.

Employing medical care in the characteristically ambivalent manner sketched above – to care for some of the patient's needs and at the same time to oppress him – is not a new phenomenon encountered first in the Soviet Union. It existed previously in Tsarist Russia as well as in Western Europe. The severity of life in Tsarist prisons – and perhaps in jails everywhere – was mitigated to some extent by the ministrations of a relatively benevolent medical personnel, the latter constituting an integral part of the prison system (see Dostoevsky, 1861–2). Since this social arrangement is widespread, I believe we are justified in placing a far-reaching interpretation on it. It may be regarded as a typical manifestation of tension in an oppressive-coercive social system, such as occurs, for example, in an autocratic-patriarchal family. In such a family, the father is a tyrant, cruelly punitive towards his children, superior and deprecatory towards his wife. The children's life is made tolerable only by the protections of a kind, devoted mother. The social pressures of the Soviet state, demanding ever-greater productivity, are reminiscent of the role of the harsh father; the citizen is the child; the protective mother is the physician.

In such a system, the mother (physician) not only protects the child (citizen) from the father (state), but, by virtue of her interventions, is also responsible for maintaining a precarious family homeostasis (or social *status quo*). To contribute to the overt breakdown of such a balance may be a constructive – and sometimes even an indispensable – step, provided that a change in the social system is considered desirable.

The Soviet medical arrangement also represents a dramatic re-enactment, in the framework of the existing social situation, of the basic human problem of dealing with 'good' and 'bad' objects. The crudely patriarchal family structure, so well described by Erikson (1950), offers a simple but highly effective solution for this problem. Instead of fostering the synthesis of love and hate for the same persons, with subsequent recognition of the complexities of human relationships, the arrangement permits and even encourages the child – and later the adult – to live in a world of devils and saints: the father is all-bad, the mother all-good. This, in turn, leads the (grown) child to feel torn between saintly righteousness and abysmal guilt. In the Soviet medical scheme, this problem and its solution appear in a new edition, as it were. The Soviet state – or better, the principles of the ideal communist system – remain the perfect 'good object'. The state furnishes *free* medical care to everyone who needs it, and the care is supposed to be *faultless*. If it is not, the blame lies with the physician. To some extent the physician thus fills the role of the 'bad object' in the Soviet social scheme.[2] The citizen (patient, child) may be viewed as being caught between the bad doctor (father) and the good state (mother). It is consistent with this thesis that the state gives much space to public accusations against doctors (Field, 1957, pp. 176–7). Although these complaints may be loud, one wonders how effective they are. Presumably the patient cannot avail himself of the protection provided for him in Western countries – the right to bring suit for malpractice against the physician. To do this would mean bringing suit against the Soviet government itself. The arrangement, however, serves well as a means to keep both patients and physicians in line. Each possesses enough power to make life difficult for the other, yet neither has sufficient freedom to alter his own situation.

In this connection, it is significant that Russian citizens who have fled their country because of dissatisfaction with the system have expressed a marked preference for Soviet medicine as against the health care patterns of West Germany and the United States (Inkeles and Bauer, 1959). Here is a striking illustration of how effectively the 'good' and 'bad' aspects of the Soviet social system have remained isolated in the minds of these people. The Soviet government's official concern for health (not specifically defined) is an unquestioned, absolute value. If something in relation to it goes wrong, another part of the system – in this case, the physician – is blamed.

The roots of the physician's role as 'social worker' can be traced to antiquity. The fusion of priestly and medical functions

[2] The famous 'doctors' plot' of early 1953 lends support to this hypothesis. It was alleged that a group of highly placed physicians murdered several key Soviet officials and were also responsible for Stalin's rapidly declining health. After Stalin's death, the plot was branded a fabrication. My point is that, irrespective of the political conflicts and motives that might have triggered this accusation, physicians – the erstwhile co-architects of the Soviet state – were now accused of destroying the very edifice they had been commissioned to build.

made for a strong bond which was split asunder only in recent times – then to be reunited, explicitly in Christian Science, implicitly in some aspects of charity practice, psychotherapy, and Soviet medicine. It is alleged that the great Virchow said: 'The physicians are the *natural attorneys of the poor*' (Field, 1957, p. 159). This concept of the physician's role must be scrutinized and challenged. There is nothing natural about it, nor is it at all clear that it is necessarily always desirable that doctors should act as though they were attorneys.

At this point, some connections between the foregoing considerations and the historical narrative concerning Charcot, presented earlier, may be noted. It was suggested that the change from diagnosing some persons as malingerers to diagnosing them as hysterics was not a medical act, but rather an act of social promotion. Charcot, too, had acted as an 'attorney for the poor'. Since that time, however, social developments in Western countries have resulted in the creation of social organizations whose duty is to be 'attorneys for the poor' (i.e. to act as representatives of their special interests). The Marxist-socialist movement itself was perhaps the first of these. There were many others, too, such as labour unions, religious organizations (which, incidentally, are the traditional guardians of the 'poor'), social work agencies, private philanthropies, and so forth. In the social setting of contemporary democracies, the physician may have a multitude of duties, but being the protector of the poor and oppressed is hardly one of them. The poor and downtrodden have their own – more or less adequate, as the case may be – representatives, at least in contemporary America. There is the National Association for the Advancement of Coloured People, the Anti-Defamation League, the Salvation Army, and a legion of other less well-known organizations whose chief purpose is the protection of various minority groups against social injustice. If we value explicitness and honesty in such matters, then this is all to the good. If an individual or group wishes to act in behalf of the interests of the poor, the Negro, the Jew, the immigrant, etc., it is desirable that this be made clear. By what right and reason, then, do physicians project themselves (*as* physicians) into the role of protectors of this or that group? Among contemporary physicians, it is the psychiatrist who, more than any other specialist, has arrogated to himself the role of protector of the downtrodden.

Concurrently with the development of appropriate social roles and institutions for the protection of the poor, the medical profession witnessed the development of many new diagnostic and therapeutic techniques. Hence, for two important reasons, it became unnecessary for the physician to function as an 'attorney for the poor'. Firstly, the poor now had real attorneys of their own, and therefore no longer needed to 'cheat' their way to being humanely treated by means of faking illness. Secondly, as the technical task which the physician had to perform became more difficult – that is, as modern surgery, pharmaco-therapy, radiology, psychotherapy, etc., came into being – the physician's role became increasingly better defined by the nature of the technical operations in which he was engaged. For example, radiologists have certain well-defined jobs, as do urologists and neurosurgeons. This being the case, they may have neither time for nor interest in the task of also acting as 'attorneys for the poor'.

A Summing Up

The prevalence of malingering in Russia, and of mental illness in the West, may be regarded as signs of the prevailing social conditions. These diagnostic labels refer only partly to the patients to whom they ostensibly point. They refer primarily to the labeller as an individual and a member of society. 'Malingering' is a manifestation of strain in a collectivistic society. The label also betrays the physician's basic identification with the values of the group. 'Mental illness', on the other hand, may be viewed as a manifestation of strain in an individualistic society. Yet mental illness is not the antonym of malingering, for the former diagnosis does not imply that the physician functions as the patient's sole agent. Mental illness is an ambiguous label. Those who use it seem to wish to straddle and evade the conflict of interests between the patient and his social environment (relatives, society, etc.). The significance of interpersonal and social conflicts tends to be obscured by emphasis on conflicts among internal objects (or identifications, roles, etc.) within the

85

patient. I do not wish to minimize the theoretical significance and psychotherapeutic value of the basic psychoanalytic position concerning the function of internal objects. My thesis is simply that it is as possible for a person to use intrapersonal conflicts (or past misfortunes) to avoid facing up to interpersonal and socio-political difficulties as it is for him to use the latter difficulties to avoid facing up to the former. It is in this connection that mental illness plays an important role as a concept that claims to explain, whereas it only explains away. This evasion of interpersonal and moral conflicts by means of the concept of mental illness is revealed by the current 'dynamic-psychiatric' view of American life (Szasz, 1960c), according to which virtually every human problem – from personal unhappiness and marital discord to political conflict and deviant moral conviction – is regarded as a symptom of mental illness.

The Historical Background

Freud's studies under Charcot centred on the problem of hysteria. When he returned to Vienna in 1886 and settled down to establish a practice in so-called nervous diseases, a large proportion of his clientele consisted of cases of hysteria (Jones, 1953). Then, even as today, the hysterical patient presented a serious challenge to the physician whom she consulted. The comfortable and safe course lay in adhering to traditional medical attitudes and procedures. This meant that the patient as a person, though the object of sympathy, could not be also the object of scientific interest. Respectable science was interested only in afflictions of the body. *Problems of human living* – or of existence, as we might say today – were thus treated as though they were manifestations of physical illnesses. The dilemma implicit in the problem of hysteria simply could not be solved within the framework of nineteenth-century thought. Breuer and Freud's singular achievement lay in adopting an attitude towards neurotic suffering that was at once humane and inquiring, compassionate and critical. Accordingly, their observations merit the closest possible attention – bearing in mind, however, that most present-day physicians and psychiatrists practise under entirely different circumstances.

It is often stated that psychoanalysts no longer encounter the type of 'hysterical illness' described by Breuer, Freud, and their contemporaries. Usually this is attributed to cultural changes, especially to the lessening of sexual repressions and to changes in the social roles of women. In addition to these factors pertaining to the position of the patient, the social role of the physician who sees hysteria has also changed. Thus while it is true that psychoanalysts, in their private offices, rarely if ever encounter 'classical cases of hysteria', this type of disability still comes to

the attention of other physicians – for example, general practitioners and various specialists in large medical centres (Ziegler
et al., 1960). I believe that hysteria, as described by Breuer and
Freud, is still prevalent in America as well as in Europe. Those
who 'suffer' from it, however, do not as a rule consult psychiatrists or psychoanalysts. Rather, they consult their family
physicians or internists and are then referred to neurologists,
neurosurgeons, orthopaedic and general surgeons, and other
medical specialists. These physicians rarely define such a
patient's difficulty as psychiatric. For that would require of
them redefining the patient's 'illness' as personal rather than
medical, something they are, understandably, not eager to
do.

Physicians also fear missing an 'organic diagnosis'. They tend
to distrust psychiatry and psychiatrists, and find it difficult to
understand what psychotherapists do. These are the main
reasons why hysterical patients have become rather rare in
private psychiatric practice. Finally, socio-economic considerations are also relevant in this connection. For reasons to be
discussed later, conversion hysteria tends nowadays to be an
affliction of relatively uneducated, lower-class persons. Hence,
they are encountered least often in the private offices of psychoanalysts – and most often in free or low-cost clinics or in state
hospitals. The few hysterics who do finally consult a psychotherapist will have had so many medical and surgical experiences
that they will no longer communicate in the pure language of
'classical hysteria'.

A Re-examination of the Data

Breuer and Freud cited examples of patients complaining of
various bodily feelings (usually of an unpleasant nature) and
then seriously complicated the issue by speaking of these
symptoms as if they constituted disorders in the physico-chemical
machinery of the human body. The following excerpt[1] illustrates
this contention:

[1] All passages cited in this chapter, unless otherwise noted, are from
Breuer and Freud's *Studies on Hysteria* (1893-5).

A highly intelligent man was present while his brother had an ankylosed hip-joint extended under an anaesthetic. At the instant at which the joint gave way with a crack, he felt a violent pain in his own hip-joint, which persisted for nearly a year. Further instances could be quoted. In other cases, the connection is not so simple. It consists only in what might be called a 'symbolic' relation between the precipitating cause and the pathological phenomenon – a relation such as healthy people form in dreams. For instance, a *neuralgia* may follow upon *mental pain* or *vomiting* upon a feeling of *moral disgust*. We have studied patients who used to make the most copious use of this sort of symbolization. ([Italics added] p. 5)

The terms 'neuralgia', 'mental pain' and 'moral disgust' refer not to observations but to complex inferences at best or philosophical preconceptions at worst. 'Neuralgia' implies a neurological, that is, physicochemical, disorder of the body. Presumably, the authors meant to say 'neuralgialike', implying that to the contemporary physician such pain suggested 'neuralgia'.

The concept of 'mental pain', like 'moral disgust', codifies the Cartesian dualism, according to which the world consists of two sets of realities, one physical, the other mental. Thus 'moral disgust' presumably must be contrasted with 'physical disgust', such as one might feel when confronted with spoiled food. But, in either case, as affects there are no discernible differences between the two. In other words, the adjective 'moral' qualifies a theoretical construct. 'Moral', 'gastrointestinal', and other possible types of disgust are, emphatically, not things any one can observe (Szasz, 1957a).

What Kind of Disease Does the Patient Have?

The crux of the difficulty which Freud faced, and to which I am pointing here, was that he was forced to ask himself the question: *What kind of disease* does this patient (who has consulted me) have? Stating the question in this form precludes the answer that he has *no disease*. Freud solved the problem by making a 'differential diagnosis', as behoved a physician. The patient's complaints are viewed as the symptoms of his (or her) particular disease.

By way of illustration, consider the following excerpt from Freud's account of the case of Fräulein Elizabeth von R.:

In the autumn of 1892, I was asked by a doctor I knew to examine a young lady who had been suffering for more than two years from pains in her legs and who had *difficulties in walking*. *All that was apparent* was that she *complained* of great pain in walking and of being quickly overcome by fatigue both in walking and in standing, and that after a short time she had to rest, which lessened the pains but did not do away with them altogether ... I did not find it easy to arrive at a *diagnosis*, but I decided for two reasons to *assent* to the one proposed by my colleague, viz., that it was a *case of hysteria*. ([Italics added] pp. 135, 136)

It was a hard fact of life that Freud was frequently faced with the need to make a differential diagnosis. He was very proud when he made a correct neurological diagnosis in a case referred to him as one of hysteria (Freud, 1905a, pp. 16–17).

Although Freud regarded hysteria as a disease, he comprehended far more, even at this early date, than could be fitted into this semantic and epistemological straitjacket. The following statement is significant in this connection:

Here, then, was the unhappy story of this proud girl with her longing for love. Unreconciled to her fate, embittered by the failure of all her little schemes for reestablishing the family's former glories, with those she loved dead or gone away or estranged, unready to take refuge in the love of some unknown man – she had lived for eighteen months in almost complete seclusion, with *nothing to occupy her but the care of her mother and her own pains*. ([Italics added] pp. 143–4)

Is this a *disease* which Freud described here? Perhaps his contemporary critics were correct when they complained that Freud did not concern himself with the same sorts of problems as did they. They recognized that Freud did not really speak about diseases of organisms (or bodies), as was then customary. Instead, he addressed himself to the problems of people as human beings, as members of society, or simply as persons.

In the passage cited above Freud spoke of an unhappy young woman and the *bodily feelings* with which she *communicated* her unhappiness. He asserted that his work was similar to the biographer's rather than to the physician's (Breuer and Freud, 1893–5, pp. 160–61). Psychoanalytic therapy rested on the assumption that the biographee would profit from a closer acquaintance with his own life history. This was a significant assumption, although by no means a novel one. The roots of this attitude to life are traceable to the ancient Greeks. The Socratic assertion that 'The unexamined life is not worth living' is the philosophy that underlies psychoanalysis as a moral and psychotherapeutic system. The maxim 'Know thyself' is the guiding rule of psychoanalytic treatment.

My thesis, then, is that Breuer and Freud's observations on hysteria, though couched in medical-psychiatric terms, are statements concerning certain patterns of human communication. Adhering closely to observations rather than to theories, we could say that the patients described were unhappy or troubled, and that they expressed their distress in so-called bodily symptoms which to the contemporary physician suggested neurological illnesses. In no case was there any evidence that the (hysterical) patient did, in fact, suffer from an anatomical or physiological disorder. Unfortunately, this did not deter Breuer and Freud from entertaining an 'organic' hypothesis for the 'cause' of this 'disease'.

A Re-examination of the Theory

Despite the novelty of some of their claims, the philosophical orientation – or, more precisely, the metascientific position – which underlay Breuer and Freud's scientific thinking was anything but unorthodox. Indeed, both men were imbued with and committed to the contemporary scientific Weltanschauung. According to it, science was synonymous with physics and chemistry (mathematics then being regarded as an auxiliary tool of these sciences). There was a tendency to force psychology into behaviourism or, that failing, to reduce it to its so-called physical and chemical bases. This goal of reducing psychological observations to physical explanations – or at least to 'instincts' – was espoused by Freud from the very beginning of his psychological studies, and he never relinquished it.

Both Breuer and Freud approached hysteria as if it were a disease essentially similar to (other) physicochemical disorders of the body (for example, syphilis). The main difference between the two was thought to be that the physico-chemical basis of hysteria was more elusive, and hence more difficult to detect with the methods then available. They acted and wrote, at least initially, as if they had to content themselves with working with psychological methods of observation and treatment, while they were waiting for the discovery of a physicochemical test of hysteria and its appropriate organic treatment. It is pertinent to recall that when *Studies on Hysteria* was published (1895), the Wasserman test had not yet been devised, and proof of the syphilitic aetiology of general paresis had not yet been histologically documented. The prevalent attitude towards psychopathology was – as it often still is – that the detection of physicochemical disorders in the human bodily machinery is the proper task facing the investigating physician. All else is an inferior substitute and must be relegated to a second-class position. Thus, psychology and psychoanalysis were given only second-class citizenship in the land of science, their emancipation remaining contingent on the discovery of a physicochemical basis of 'mind' and behaviour.

This search for the physical causation of so-called psychopathological phenomena is motivated more by a need for prestige on the part of the investigators than by a quest for scientific clarity. We touched on a related issue when it was suggested that adherence to the medical model of thought enables the psychiatrist to share in the prestige of the physician's role. We encounter here the same phenomenon with respect to the prestige of the investigator or research worker. Since investigators in physics enjoy greater prestige than those in psychology or in the study of human relations, it is advantageous for psychiatrists and psychoanalysts to claim that, fundamentally, they too search for physical or physiological causes of bodily illness. This makes them, of course, pseudo-physicists and pseudo-physicians, and has many regrettable consequences. Yet, this striving for prestige by imitating the natural scientist has also been successful, at least in a social or opportunistic way. By 'success' I refer to the widespread social acceptance of psychiatry and psychoanalysis as allegedly biological (and hence ultimately physicochemical) *sciences*, and to the prestige of their practitioners based, in part, on this connection between what they claim they do and what other (physical) scientists do.

Freud's original concept of hysterical conversion was stated concisely in the following lines (apropos of the case of Fräulein Elizabeth von R.):

According to the view suggested by the conversion theory of hysteria, what happened may be described as follows: *She repressed her erotic idea from consciousness and transformed the amount of its affect into physical sensations of pain.* ([Italics added] p. 164)

This theory calls for closer examination. We may ask: What is it that turns into physical pain here? A cautious reply would be: Something that might have become, and should have become, *mental pain.* If we venture a little further and try to represent the ideational mechanism in a kind of algebraical picture, we may attribute a certain quota of affect to the ideational complex of these erotic feelings which remained unconscious, and say that *this quantity* (the quota of affect) *is what was converted.* ([Italics added] p. 166)

Here we have the problem of conversion hysteria in *statu nascendi*. Freud asked: What is being converted (to physical pain)? Why does the patient *have* physical pain? Ancillary questions are: What causes it? How does a conflict, or affect, become converted to physical pain?

Freud replied by taking recourse to what Colby (1955) aptly called a 'hydraulic metaphor'. It seems evident, however, that no such complicated explanation is required. All that is necessary is to frame our questions differently. We might then ask: Why does a patient *complain* of pain? Ancillary questions are: Why does the patient complain about his body when it is physically intact? Why does the patient not complain about personal troubles? If we ask the second set of questions, then the answers must be phrased in terms of the complainant's personal troubles. Actually, Breuer and Freud's descriptions of their patients go far in answering these questions.

Let us see just how much the idea of hysterical complaints *as symptoms* of physical (bodily) disorders has complicated our problem. Freud wrote:

The mechanism was that of conversion: i.e., in place of *mental pains* which she avoided, *physical pains* made their appearance. In this way a transformation was effected which had the advantage that the patient escaped from an intolerable *mental condition*: though, it is true, this was at the cost of a *psychical abnormality* – the splitting of consciousness that came about, and of a *physical illness* – her pains, in which an astasia-abasia was built up. ([Italics added] p. 166)

Throughout this passage – and it is illustrative of many others – the words 'mental' and 'physical' appear as if they described observations, when in fact they are theoretical concepts used to order and 'explain' the observations. On the basis of Freud's foregoing definition of conversion, it would be justifiable to assert that the problem is epistemological rather than psychiatric. In other words, *there is no problem of conversion, unless we insist on so framing our questions that we inquire about physical disorders where, in fact, none exist.*

In effect, Freud asked: Why does a psychological problem take physical form? How does a psychological problem become manifest as a physical phenomenon? These questions recodified the classic riddle of the 'jump from the psychic into the organic' which psychoanalysis, and especially the theory of conversion, then sought to elucidate. Because of this conceptual framework, so-called psychological phenomena – such as bodily complaints, and so-called physical phenomena – such as anatomical or bio-chemical alterations, have been juxtaposed as if they constituted two sides of the same coin.

I believe that this view is completely false. We shall not regard the relationship between the psychological and the physical as a relationship between two different types of events or occur-rences, but shall rather consider it to be akin to two different modes of representation or language (Russell, 1948).

I submit that the classical models of hysteria and conversion are no longer useful either for nosology or for therapy. Today, however, there may be social and institutional grounds for adhering to this theory. The notion of hysteria as mental illness, and the psychoanalytic theory of hysteria (especially the idea of conversion), have become the symbols of psychoanalysis as a medical technique and guild. The original psychoanalytic theory of hysteria – and of neurosis, following more or less closely on the same scheme – made it possible for physicians (and allied scientists) to retain a fairly homogeneous picture of 'diseases'. According to this scheme, diseases could be divided into somatic and psychical; and psychotherapy could be regarded as an enterprise essentially similar to established modes of medical and surgical treatments. The alternative to this familiar and comfortable point of view is to abandon the entire physicalistic-medical approach to mental illness and to substitute novel theoretical viewpoints and models, appropriate to psychological, social, and ethical problems. Explicit recognition of the social (institutional) function of certain present-day psychiatric ideas and practices should prove helpful in an analysis of the roots of the notion of mental illness.

5 Contemporary Views on Hysteria and Mental Illness

Although a newcomer among the professions and sciences, psychiatry is characterized by a plethora of diverse, competing, and often mutually exclusive theories and practices. Actually, psychiatry is more like religion and politics than science. In religion and politics we expect to find conflicting systems or ideologies. Widespread consensus concerning the practical management of human affairs, and the ethical systems utilized in governing and justifying particular types of group formations, are regarded merely as indices of the political success of the governing ideology. Matters of scientific theory (and, to some extent, also of scientific practice) do not as a rule concern vast populations. Hence, large-scale consensus in regard to such matters is not expected. At the same time, it is unusual for scientists widely and persistently to disagree among themselves concerning the explanations and practices appropriate to their special areas of competence. For instance, there is, as a rule, little disagreement among scientists concerning basic physiological, biochemical, or physical theories – even though individual scientists may believe in different religions (or in no religion) and may be members of different national groups. This is not true for psychiatry.

In studying human behaviour, we are confronted by the disconcerting fact that psychiatric theories are nearly as numerous and varied as psychiatric symptoms. This is true not only in historical and international perspectives but also within single nations. Thus, it is especially difficult to describe and compare, say, American and English, or American and Swiss psychiatry, for none of these countries presents a psychiatrically united front. The reasons for this state of affairs, and its important implications for our efforts to build an internationally respectable science of psychiatry, cannot be considered here. I should like to emphasize only that I believe that much of the difficulty in the way of building a coherent theory of human behaviour lies in our inability – sometimes unwillingness – to separate *description from prescription*. Such questions as 'How *are* men constituted?' 'How *do* they act?' 'What *are* the relations between society and the individual?' can and must be separated from such questions as 'How *should* men act?' or 'What *should* be the relations between society and the individual?'

Psychoanalytic Conceptions

Fenichel (1945), the author of a highly respected psychoanalytic text, distinguished anxiety hysteria from conversion hysteria. Anxiety hysteria, which is also a synonym for phobia, he described as the 'simplest compromise between drive and defence' (p. 194); the anxiety motivating the defence becomes manifest, while the 'reason for the anxiety' remains repressed. In other words, the person experiences anxiety without knowing why. Fenichel illustrated this process by citing the example of 'Small children [who] are afraid of being left alone, which for them means not being loved any more' (p. 196). The psychology of anxiety hysteria is laid bare here as simply a connection, on the part of the child, between the experiences of being left alone and being unloved. Since it is considered normal for children to feel anxious when they are unloved, this reaction is not defined as a psychological disease entity. However, being left alone, by itself, is not considered a sufficient cause for feeling anxious. Hence, if such a reaction occurs, it must be due to something else. The *meaning* of being left alone is then advanced as the *cause* of the 'abnormal reaction' called a 'phobia'.

The child's experience of anxiety on being left alone may be interpreted in at least two ways. Firstly, it may be considered pathological (or 'bad') if it is assumed that the reaction signifies excessive proneness to feeling unloved (perhaps because of many actual experiences of rejection). Secondly, the reaction may be considered normal (or 'good') if it is regarded as an expression of the child's ability to learn and symbolize, and hence make

97

connections between superficially more or less dissimilar situations. According to the latter view, a phobia, and virtually all other 'psychopathological symptoms', are similar to scientific hypotheses. Both types of phenomena – that is, 'making mental symptoms' as well as making hypotheses – rest on the fundamental human tendency to construct symbolic representations and use them to guide subsequent behaviour.

In his discussion of conversion hysteria, Fenichel (1945) consistently used the mixed physical and psychological language which I have criticized earlier. For example, he spoke of 'physical functions' providing unconscious expression for repressed 'instinctual impulses' (p. 216). Here, just as in Breuer and Freud's writings, complaints about the body ('hysterical pain') or communications by means of bodily behaviour (gestures, 'hysterical paralysis') were erroneously described as alterations in physical functions. I believe that the crux of the matter is simply that in conversion hysteria the symptom refers to the patient's body, whereas in anxiety hysteria it points to a human situation (loneliness in a dark room).

The significance of unrecognized epistemological errors in the concept of hysteria may be illustrated by Fenichel's following analysis of a case of so-called hysterical pain:

A patient suffered from pain in the lower abdomen. The pain repeated sensations she had felt as a child during an attack of appendicitis. At that time she had been treated with unusual tenderness by her father. *The abdominal pain expressed simultaneously a longing for the father's tenderness and a fear that an even more painful operation might follow a fulfilment of this longing.* ([Italics added] p. 220)

In contrast, consider an account of the same type of phenomenon as described by Woodger (1956). It concerns the case of a girl who developed abdominal pain and consulted a surgeon.

He [i.e., the surgeon] recommended an operation for the removal of the appendix and this was accordingly performed. But after recovery and convalescence the girl again complained of abdominal pain. This time she was advised to consult a surgeon with a view to treatment for adhesions resulting from the first operation. But the second surgeon referred the girl to a psychiatrist from whose inquiries it transpired that the girl's education had been such that she believed it to be possible to become pregnant by being kissed. The first abdominal pain had appeared after the experience of being kissed by an undergraduate during his vacation. After the recovery from the operation this girl was again kissed by the same undergraduate with a similar result. (p. 57)

In the psychoanalytic formulation of the *observational datum* (abdominal pain), there is a constant intrusion of abstractions expressing the preformed philosophical attitudes of the observer. Thus, Fenichel spoke (in an earlier passage not quoted) of the 'original physical pain', and contrasted it with the current, presumably 'hysterical pain'. He then proceeded to translate 'abdominal pain' into a 'longing for the father's tenderness'. Thus, the crucial issue of validation was completely omitted. In other words, could it not happen that the patient's abdominal pain was *caused*, say, by tubal pregnancy, and that it also *meant* that she longed for her father's love?

The problem of whether the 'meaning' of pain could also be its 'cause', and if so in what way, is far more complicated than the psychoanalytic theory of hysteria would have it. According to the latter, some pains are 'organic', others 'hysterical'. Thus a longing, a wish, a need – broadly speaking, psychological 'meanings' of all sorts – are regarded as 'causal agents' similar, in all significant respects, to tumours, fractures, and other bodily lesions. Clearly, nothing could be more misleading, since fractures and tumours belong in one logical class, while desires, aspirations, and conflicts belong in another (Ryle, 1949). I am not saying that psychological motives can never be regarded as 'causes' of human conduct, for evidently this is often a useful way of describing social behaviour. It should be kept in mind, however, that my desire to see a play is the 'cause' of my going to the theatre in a sense very different from that in which we speak of 'causal laws' in physics (Peters, 1958).

Glover (1949), too, followed the usual psychiatric classification in regard to hysteria. He asserted that 'two major types of hysteria exist, namely, conversion hysteria and anxiety hysteria' (p. 140). He thus implied that 'hysteria' is an entity found in nature rather than an abstraction or theoretical construct made by man. Moreover, he too employed a mixed physical and psychological language – for example, in speaking of 'physical symptoms' and 'psychic contents'. Thus, the above-mentioned criticisms apply to his writings as well.

However, one of Glover's formulations was novel and deserves special comment. It is the notion, today widely accepted by psychoanalysts, that conversion symptoms possess 'specific psychic content', whereas so-called psychosomatic symptoms do not (pp. 140–41). This distinction, useful as it is, could be formulated more simply by comparing the former to actions, and the latter to happenings. In other words, conversion symptoms are intentional signs: they are bits of behaviour that are intended to convey a message. This is why they must be regarded as communications. In contrast, so-called psychosomatic symptoms – say, peptic ulcer or diarrhoea – are in the nature of physical (pathophysiological) occurrences. As such, they are not intended to be communications. Nevertheless, they may be interpreted as signs by certain observers (who may be astute and knowledgeable, or stupid and mistaken, as the case may be). Accordingly, psychosomatic symptoms (of this type) – much as happenings of all sorts – need not be looked upon as communications. However, since *not all communications are intentional*, psychosomatic symptoms, too, may validly be interpreted as messages of a certain type.

This point of view is, indeed, implicit in the classic psychoanalytic papers of Freud and Ferenczi. The communicational possibilities of diseases of all types (and not only of a few specially labelled as 'psychosomatic'), for both diagnosis and treatment, inspired Groddeck (1927, 1934) to propose far-reaching, and at times fantastic, interpretations of these phenomena. Groddeck's ideas, though scientifically unsystematized and unverified, must be considered forerunners of subsequent developments which led to a better appreciation of the communicational significance of all human behaviour.

Beginning in the 1930s, psychoanalysts began to place increasing emphasis on so-called ego-psychology – which meant, among other things, emphasis on communicative, interpersonal behaviour rather than on instinctual needs and their vicissitudes. At about the same time, Sullivan provided impetus for an explicitly interpersonal – sociologic and communicational – approach to psychiatry and especially to psychotherapy. He thus spearheaded a trend that has become general within the body of psychoanalysis itself. I refer to the increasingly explicit recognition that human experiences and relationships – and especially human communications – are the most significant observables with which psychoanalysts and psychosocially oriented psychiatrists deal.

Although I consider Sullivan's contribution to psychiatry impressive, many of his early theoretical formulations – especially those concerning so-called psychiatric syndromes – were modifications of, rather than improvements on, Freud's ideas. For example, in *Conceptions of Modern Psychiatry* (1947), Sullivan proposed this definition of hysteria:

Hysteria, the mental disorder to which the self-absorbed are peculiarly liable, is the distortion of inter-personal relations which results from extensive amnesias. (p. 54)

Sullivan's description of hysterical strategies, though unencumbered by physiologizing about behaviour, is open to the same criticisms as were levelled against the traditional psychoanalytic concept. For Sullivan, too, spoke of hysteria as though it were a disease entity. And he believed that amnesias caused this disorder. But how could amnesia 'cause' hysteria? Is this not like saying that fever 'causes' pneumonia? Moreover, Sullivan's formulation was only a modification of Freud's (1910a) classic dictum that 'hysterical patients suffer from reminiscences' (p. 16).

There can be little doubt, of course, that both Freud and Sullivan were correct in identifying painful ('traumatic') memories, their repression, and their persistent operation as significant antecedents in the personal and social behaviour of hysterically disabled individuals. In his later work, Sullivan (1956) described hysteria as a form of communication and laid the ground for viewing it as a special type of game-playing behaviour. His views on hysteria will be discussed again in connection with the presentation of a game-model theory of this phenomenon (Chapter 14).

Fairbairn (1952) has been one of the most successful exponents of a consistently psychological formulation of psychiatric problems. Emphasizing that psychoanalysis deals with observations of, and statements about, 'object relationships' (that is, human relationships), he has reformulated much of psychoanalytic theory from the vantage point of this ego-psychological (and, by implication, communicational) approach. In his paper, 'Observations on the Nature of Hysterical States' (1954), he wrote:

Hysterical conversion is, of course, a defensive technique – one designed to prevent the conscious emergence of emotional conflicts involving object-relationships. Its essential and distinctive feature *is the substitution of a bodily state for a personal problem*; and this substitution enables the personal problem as such to be ignored. (p. 117)

I am in agreement with this simple yet precise statement. According to it, the distinctive feature of hysteria is the substitution of a 'bodily state' for communications by means of ordinary language concerning personal problems. As a result of this transformation both the content and the form of the discourse change. The content changes from personal problems to bodily problems, while the form changes from verbal (linguistic) language to bodily (gestural) language.

Accordingly, *hysterical conversion is best regarded as a process of translation* – a conception first proposed by Freud. It was Sullivan and Fairbairn, however, who gave impetus to the fuller appreciation of the communicative aspects of all types of occurrences encountered in psychiatric and psychotherapeutic work.

Organic Theories

No attempt will be made to review the principal organic – that is, biochemical, genetic, pathophysiological, etc. – theories of hysteria. I shall only state my position vis-à-vis organic theories of hysteria (and mental illness, generally) and their relation to the present work.

Many physicians, psychiatrists, psychologists, and other scientists believe that mental diseases have organic causes. Let me make clear that I do not contend that human relations, or mental events, take place in a neurophysiological vacuum. It is more than likely that if a person, say an Englishman, decides to study French, certain chemical (or other) changes will occur in his brain as he learns the language. Nevertheless, I think it would be a mistake to infer from this assumption that the most significant or useful statements about this learning process must be expressed in the language of physics. This, however, is exactly what the organicist claims.

Notwithstanding the widespread social acceptance of psychoanalysis in contemporary America, there remains a wide circle of physicians and allied scientists whose basic position concerning the problem of mental illness is essentially that expressed in Carl Wernicke's famous dictum: 'Mental diseases are brain diseases'. Because, in one sense, this is true of such conditions as paresis (and the psychoses associated with brain tumour or systematic intoxications), it is argued that it is also true for all other things *called* mental diseases. It follows that it is only a matter of time until the correct physico-chemical, including genetic, bases (or 'causes') of these disorders will be discovered (e.g. Pauling, 1956). It is conceivable, of course, that significant physiochemical disturbances will be found in some patients (and 'conditions') now loosely labelled mental illnesses. But this does not mean that all so-called mental diseases have biological 'causes', for the simple reason that it has become customary to use the term 'mental illness' to stigmatize, and thus control, those persons whose behaviour offends society (or the psychiatrist making the 'diagnosis').

Let us sharply distinguish between two epistemological positions. The first, extreme physicalism, asserts that only physics and its branches can be considered sciences (J. R. Weinberg, 1950). Hence, all observations must be formulated in the language of physics. The second position, a sort of liberal empiricism, recognizes a variety of legitimate methods and languages within the family of science (Mises, 1951). Indeed, since different types of problems are considered to require different methods of analysis, a diversity of scientific methods and expressions (languages) is not merely tolerated but is rather considered a *sine qua non* of science. According to this position, the value, and hence the scientific legitimacy, of any particular method or language depends on its pragmatic utility, rather than on how closely it approximates the ideal model of theoretical physics.

It is well to recognize that both of these attitudes towards science rest on certain value judgements. Physicalism (and variations on its theme) asserts that all of the sciences should, as far as possible, be like physics. If we adhere to this view, the physical (which, in the case of medicine, includes the chemical, physiological, etc.) bases of human performances will be regarded as most significant. In contrast, the second type of scientific attitude (whether it is called empiricism, pragmatism, operationism, or by some other name) focuses on the value of instrumental utility – that is, the power to explain the observed and to influence it.

It seems to me that most of those who adhere to an organicist position in psychiatry espouse a system of values of which they are unaware. They imply that they recognize as scientific only physics (and its branches), but instead of asserting this clearly and explicitly, they say that they object to psychosocial theories only because they are false. Here is a typical example:

From the results of this investigation, it seems proper to suggest that the *diagnosis* of hysteria might be made by following the *standard procedure* used in the general field of *diagnostic medicine*: that is, determining the facts of the chief complaint, past history, physical examination and laboratory investigation. If the relevant symptoms of hysteria are known, this method can be applied by *any physician* without the use of special techniques, dream analysis or prolonged investigation of *psychological conflicts*. These studies give no information about the *cause* of hysteria or about the specific mechanisms of symptoms. *It is believed that these are unknown.* Further, it is believed that they will be discovered by *scientific* investigation, rather than by the use of *non-scientific methods*, such as pure discussion, speculation, further reasoning from the dictums of 'authorities' or 'schools of psychology' or by the use of such pretentious undefined words as 'unconscious', 'depth psychology', 'psychodynamics', 'psycho-somatic', and 'Oedipus complex' and that fundamental investigation must rest on a firm *clinical basis*. ([Italics added] Purtell *et al.*, 1951, p. 909)

I hope that the authors' complaints against psychoanalysis will not distract the reader from noting that they have defined science covertly so as to exclude the nonphysical disciplines from it.

In short, we may conclude that the psychologically minded psychiatrist and his organicist colleague, though often members of the same professional organizations, do not talk the same language and do not have the same interests. It is not surprising, then, that they have nothing to say to each other, and that when they do communicate it is only to castigate each other's work and point of view.

BOOK TWO
Foundations of a Theory of
Personal Conduct

PART II
Semiotical Analysis of Behaviour

6   Language and Protolanguage

The definitions of such terms as 'language', 'sign', and 'symbol' will be indispensable for our further work.[1] The concept of sign is the most basic of the three, and we shall start with it. Signs are, first of all, physical things: for example, chalk marks on a blackboard, pencil or ink marks on paper, sound waves produced in a human throat. 'What makes them signs,' according to Reichenbach (1947), 'is the intermediary position they occupy between an object and a sign user, i.e. a person' (p. 4). For a sign to be a sign, or to function as such, it is necessary that the person take account of the object it designates. Thus, *anything in nature may or may not be a sign, depending on a person's attitude towards it*. A physical thing is a sign when it appears as a substitute for, or representation of, the object for which it stands with respect to the sign user. The three-place relation between sign, object, and sign user is called the *sign relation* or *relation of denotation*.

The Structure of Protolanguage

According to strict symbolic-logical usage, to use signs is not the same as to use language. What, then, are nonlinguistic signs? We may distinguish, still following Reichenbach, three classes of signs. In the first class may be placed signs that acquire their function through a *causal connection* between object and sign: smoke, for example, is a sign of fire. Signs of this type are called *indexical*. The second class is made up of signs that stand in a

[1] In this connection, the reader may wish to consult Reichenbach (1947), whose conceptual scheme was adopted as the basis for the present exposition.

relation of *similarity* to the objects they designate: for example, the photograph of a man or the map of a terrain. These are called *iconic signs*. In the third class are placed signs whose relation to the object is purely *conventional* or *arbitrary*: for example, words or mathematical symbols. These are called *conventional signs* or *symbols*. *Symbols* usually do not exist in isolation, but are coordinated with each other by a set of rules, called the rules of language. The entire package, consisting of symbols, language rules, and social customs concerning language use, is sometimes referred to as the *language game*. In the technical idiom of the logician, we speak of language *only* when communication is mediated by means of systematically coordinated conventional signs.

According to this definition, there can be no such thing as a 'body language'. If we wish to express ourselves precisely, we must speak instead of *communication by means of bodily signs*. This is not mere pedantry. The expression 'bodily sign' implies two significant characteristics. Firstly, that we deal here with something other than conventional, linguistic symbols. Secondly, that the signs in question must be identified further as to their special characteristics. In speaking of bodily signs, I shall always refer to phenomena such as so-called hysterical paralyses, blindness, deafness, seizures, and so forth. These occurrences speak for themselves, as it were, and hence communication by means of such signs need not involve speech. In this, they are distinguished from certain other bodily signs, such as pain, which may be communicated either verbally or by pantomime (i.e. by behaviour suggesting to the observer that the sufferer is in pain). Finally, since speech itself makes use of bodily organs, it too could loosely be called a 'bodily sign'. This, however, would be a vague and non-technical use of this expression. By adhering to a more precise definition, we can readily differentiate between two types of speech: firstly, ordinary speech, *using socially shared symbols* (called language), and secondly, the use of *vocal noises that are not symbols* (e.g. schizophrenic vocalizations). The latter, although making use of the so-called speech apparatus, *logically* belongs in the same class as bodily signs. So much for initial definitions. Let us now take up the question posed earlier: What are the characteristic features of the signs employed in so-called body language?

Body Language is composed of Iconic Signs

The concept of iconic sign fits exactly the phenomena described as body signs. The relationship of iconic sign to denoted object is one of similarity. A photograph, for example, is an iconic sign of the person in the picture. Similarly, an *hysterical seizure is an iconic sign of a genuine (organic) epileptic seizure*; or, an hysterical paralysis or weakness of the lower extremities may be an iconic sign of weakness due to multiple sclerosis or tabes dorsalis. In brief, *body signs are best conceptualized as iconic signs of bodily illness*. This interpretation is consistent with the fact that communications of this type occur chiefly in interactions between a sufferer and his helper. The two participants may or may not be specifically defined as patient and physician. The point is that body signs, as iconic signs of bodily illness, form an integral part of what might best be called the *language of illness*. In other words, just as photographs as iconic signs have special relevance to the movie industry and its patrons, so iconic signs pertaining to the body have special relevance to the 'healing industry' and its patrons.

Body Language is a Protolanguage

Again, it is necessary to consider briefly the technical classification of languages devised by logicians. Philologists and linguists have classified languages in accordance with their own interests and needs. These classifications distinguish different individual languages, such as English, German, French, Hungarian, and so forth. Individual tongues and dialects are then ordered into larger groups called families of languages. Thus, we speak of Indo-European, Finno-Ugric, Indian, and other groups, in each of which many individual languages are subsumed.

Logicians and philosophers, under the impetus of Whitehead and Russell (1910), have developed a completely different kind of language classification, according to which languages are distinguished from one another depending on the level of complexity of the logical descriptions and operations involved. The first, or lowest level, is called object language.[2] The signs of this language denote physical objects, for example, cat, dog, chair, table, and so on. We may next introduce signs referring to signs. The words 'word', 'sentence', 'clause', and 'phrase' are signs belonging to (the first-level) metalanguage. This iteration of the coordination of signs and referents may be repeated *ad infinitum*. Thus, progressively higher levels of metalanguages can be constructed, by for ever introducing signs which denote signs at the next lower logical level. The distinction between object language and metalanguage (and metalanguages of increasingly higher orders) is the single most significant contribution of symbolic logic to the science of language. Only by means of this distinction did it become apparent that in order to speak about any object language, we need a metalanguage. It must be remembered, of course, that on both of these levels of language, the same linguistic stock may be used. Thus, wrote Jakobson (1957), 'we may speak in English (as metalanguage) about English (as object language) and interpret English words and sentences by means of English synonyms, circumlocutions, and paraphrases' (p. 163). So-called ordinary language consists of a mixture of object and metalanguages.

For our present purposes, it is especially important to note that, in this scheme, the lowest level of language is object language. *There is no room here for what goes in psychiatry by the name of body language.* This is because body language is composed of iconic signs. Hence, it constitutes a system logically more primitive than the operations of object language.

In as much as conventional signs (or symbols) make up the lowest level of language, and signs of signs the first level of metalanguage, and so on, a communication system employing

[2] The word 'object' is used in several different senses in this book, depending on the context in which it appears. It is used in a technically specialized fashion in two situations. In connection with object relationships, 'object' usually means a person, less often a thing or idea. In connection with logical hierarchies, say of languages, the term 'object' denotes a level of discourse about which one may speak only in a metalanguage. The logical relationship between object and meta levels is always a relative one. Thus a first-level metalanguage may be considered an object language with respect to a second-level metalanguage.

signs that denote less, as it were, than do conventional signs may be regarded as forming a level of language below that of object language. I suggest, therefore, that we call this type of (body) language a *protolanguage*. This seems fitting since the word 'metalanguage' denotes that languages of this type are later, beyond, or higher than object languages. The prefix 'proto', being the antonym of 'meta', refers to something that is earlier or lower than something else (as in 'prototype').

Placing certain types of body symptoms – that is, those that are iconic signs – in their proper places in the logical hierarchy of languages will be of considerable help in formulating psychiatric problems. To begin with, the very notion of understanding something hinges on its expressibility, either in conversational or in technical languages. This means that whatever it might be that we try to understand or describe must be expressed in terms of object and metalanguages. What, then, is the function of protolanguage? As we shall see, it is not quite true that intelligible communication is possible only by means of object and metalanguages.

The Nature of Protolinguistic Communication

An hysterical symptom, say a seizure or paralysis, expresses and transmits a message, usually to a specific person. A paralysed arm, for instance, may mean: 'I have sinned with this arm and have been punished for it.' It may also mean 'I wanted or needed to obtain some forbidden gratification (erotic, aggressive, etc.) by means of this arm.' But what exactly is meant when it is stated that a symptom has such and such a meaning? This problem raises such related questions as: does the patient – the sender of the message – know *that* he is communicating, and *what* he is communicating? Does the receiver of the message – physician, husband, wife, etc. – know *that* he or she is being communicated with, and *what* is being communicated to him or her? If they do not know these things, how can they be said to be communicating?

Although Freud never raised these questions, at least not as I have framed them, he gave some good answers to them. Perhaps precisely because they were so useful, his answers obscured the original questions which stimulated them and which were never explicitly stated. Freud suggested that we distinguish two basically different types of 'mentation' and 'knowledge', one conscious, the other unconscious. Unconscious activity is directed by so-called primary processes, while conscious mentation is logically organized and is governed by so-called secondary processes (Fenichel, 1945, pp. 14–15, 46–51).

The term 'conscious' was never specifically defined in psychoanalysis, but was used rather in a common-sense, phenomenological sense. The concept 'unconscious' was much more carefully elaborated by Freud (1915), and was later differentiated from the 'preconscious'. For our present purpose, it is enough that Freud spoke of the unconscious partly as if it were a region in the mental apparatus, and partly as if it were a system of operations. He assumed the existence of such alleged occurrences as unconscious knowledge, unconscious conflicts, unconscious needs, and so forth, and used these expressions to describe them.

Unfortunately, this terminology obscures some of the logical problems that must be solved. It is basic to science as a social enterprise that we recognize as knowledge only that which can be made public. This is why the scientific idea of knowledge – as contrasted with mystical or religious versions of it – is so inextricably tied to the notion of representation by means of conventional signs. What cannot be expressed in either object or metalanguage cannot, by definition, be knowledge. For instance, a painting may be interesting and beautiful, yet its 'meaning' cannot be called knowledge.

If we adhere to this more precise terminology it will be necessary to concede that body languages of the type considered *do not*, as such, express *knowledge*. This is not the same as to assert that they are devoid of *information*. We touch here on the distinction between knowledge and information, which, in our usage, is the same as the distinction between verbal symbol and iconic sign. Thus, a cloudy sky may be said to 'contain' information, for its 'message' could be read by a person as a sign of impending rain. We may not say, however, that a cloudy sky 'contains' knowledge. Similarly, to obtain the hidden meaning, so to speak, of a message framed in the idiom of body signs, it is necessary to translate protolanguage into ordinary language. Freud expressed a similar idea when he spoke of making the unconscious conscious, or translating the former into the latter. Yet *he never clearly conceptualized the 'unconscious' as nothing but a language or a form of communication.* Hence, while the idea of translating protolanguage into ordinary language *describes* some of the same things that Freud described as rendering the unconscious conscious, the two schemes are not identical.[3]

A question has been raised concerning the connection between the use of protolanguage and the sender's 'knowledge' of the messages so communicated. This relationship is an inverse one. In other words, while it is usually impossible to speak about something one does not know, one may readily express by means of protolanguage that which is not explicitly known or socially acknowledged. This is because learning and knowledge on the one hand, and symbolic codification and communication (language, mathematics, etc.) on the other, are interdependent and can grow only together (Szasz, 1957c). Since the use of iconic (body) signs is the simplest communicational device available to man, communication of this type varies inversely with knowledge and learning. The thesis that relatively less sophisticated persons are more likely to use protolanguage is consistent with our knowledge concerning the historical and social determinants of so-called hysterical symptoms. Consider, for example, the time when human beings tried literally to be the *icons* of Christ on the cross, exhibiting so-called hysterical stigmata. 'Conversations' in this sort of protolanguage can occur only if the participants in the communicational process do not easily speak a higher level of language. As a more sceptical attitude developed towards religion, this form of protolinguistic communication began to disappear, and was replaced by one making use of the imagery of illness and treatment.

[3] There are some similarities between what I have called *protolanguage* and Freud's concept of *primary process* thinking, and also between it and the *palaeologic* of Von Domarus and Arieti (Arieti, 1955, 1959). The differences between protolanguage and the two latter constructs should become clear in the course of the subsequent exposition.

Symbolization in Hysteria: a Critical Example

I will now illustrate my thesis by means of an excerpt from Breuer and Freud's *Studies on Hysteria* (1893–5). The following is from Freud's account of his treatment of Frau Cäcilie M.:

In this phase of the work we came at last to the reproduction of her facial neuralgia, which I myself had treated when it appeared in contemporary attacks. I was curious to discover whether this, too, would turn out to have a psychical cause. When I began to call up the traumatic scene, the patient saw herself back in a period of great mental irritability towards her husband. She described a conversation which she had with him and a remark of his which she had felt as a bitter insult. Suddenly she put her hand to her cheek, gave a loud cry of pain and said: 'It was like a slap in the face.' With this her pain and her attack were both at an end.

There is no doubt that what had happened had been a *symbolization*. She had felt as though she had actually been given a slap in the face. Everyone will immediately ask how it was that the sensation of a 'slap in the face' came to take on the outward forms of a *trigeminal neuralgia*, why it was restricted to the second and third branches, and why it was made worse by opening the mouth and chewing – though, incidentally, not by talking.

Next day the *neuralgia* was back again. But this time its was cleared up by the reproduction of another scene, the content of which was once again a supposed *insult*. Things went on like this for nine days. It seemed to be the case that *for years insults, and particularly spoken ones, had, through symbolization, brought on fresh attacks of her facial neuralgia*. ([Italics added] p. 178)

Here, as elsewhere, Freud spoke of a process of 'symbolization' by means of which an insult was transformed into pain. Freud called this 'conversion', thus perpetuating the so-called riddle of the jump from the psychic into the organic. Yet, all one needs to do is to conceptualize this in terms of translation, and the problems of conversion and psychogenesis assume novel, more manageable proportions.

I assume that at least one of the reasons for Freud's failure to carry through consistently with the model of translation was that he did not grasp exactly what type of symbolization he had identified. How can a slap on the face be 'converted' to (what looks like) trigeminal neuralgia? How can the one be a symbol for the other? Freud did not answer these questions nor, in fact, did he raise them. Instead, he proceeded as follows. First, he assumed that the symbolization described above is essentially similar to that obtaining between verbal symbol and referent. Then he proceeded as if this had been a fact, instead of an unverified – and, as it turned out, incorrect – assumption. Accordingly, he interpreted hysterical symptoms as if the translation they required were no different from, say, rendering ancient Greek into modern English. Furthermore, he approached the reason for or motives behind the symbolization through the traditional model of medicine. The problem thus became: why does 'conversion' occur? Or, stated more generally: why does a 'patient' 'develop' 'hysteria'? In this way, Freud ended up with a classic *medical* problem: namely, with the problem of the 'aetiology of hysteria'. However, if hysteria is a language, looking for its 'aetiology' is about as sensible as is looking for the 'aetiology' of mathematics. A language has a history, a geographic distribution, a system of rules for its use . . . but it does not have an 'aetiology'.

There remains for us to consider the type of symbol which Freud described in the case history cited. How can a facial pain represent a slap on the face? Why should an insult be so denoted? It appears that this type of symbolization hinges on a two-fold relation.

Firstly, there is the similarity between pain caused by a slap and pain caused by neuralgia (meaning thereby *any* physical disorder whose symptom is facial pain). Hence, Frau Cäcilie's facial pain is an iconic sign of (the pain due to) a facial illness. Indeed, to some extent every pain constitutes an iconic sign of every other. Just as in a picture of an egg we recognize every egg we ever saw, so each pain we experience is, in part, built up of all the pains we have ever had.

Secondly, the pain of a slapped face, or of being insulted and humiliated, is not only an iconic sign of facial neuralgia – it is *also* an indexical sign of it. This is because being slapped and having a pain stand in a temporal and cause-and-effect relationship to one another. We know, or can infer, 'slaps' from 'pains', even though this may not be the only way in which such information can be obtained. Hence, a pain can be an indexical sign of being slapped in the face or of having trigeminal neuralgia – in the same way as having a fever can be an indexical sign of an infection. Both types of sign-relations enter into the actual communicational patterns we are considering. For example, a woman communicating facial pain to her husband may 'sound' to him – especially if he has hurt her – as if she were saying: 'Do you see now how you have hurt me?' The same woman making the same communication to her physician may, on the other hand, 'sound' to him as if she were saying: 'I have trigeminal neuralgia.' Although both husband and physician interpret the pain as a sign at once iconic and indexical, they read it quite differently depending on their specific position in the three-place relation holding between sign, object, and interpreter of sign. It is because of his special position in this three-place relation that the psychoanalyst tends to read the facial pain as an iconic sign – that is, as: 'This looks like neuralgia but probably is not.'

There remains the question of why a slap on the face should be denoted by facial pains. It should suffice to note here – as this question will be discussed in detail in Chapter 7 – that the use of this type of body language is fostered by circumstances that make direct verbal expression difficult or impossible. The custom of referring to sexual organs and activities by Latin words rather than in one's native tongue affords a typical illustration. Translation from what could be, or had been, ordinary language into protolanguage serves a similar purpose. It makes communication about an important but delicate subject possible, while at the same time it helps the speaker disown the disturbing implications of his message. The specific choice of body signs is generally determined by the unique personal and social circumstances of the sufferer, in accordance with the principles discovered by Freud.

The Function of Protolanguage

Thus far we have considered only two aspects of the body language characteristic of so-called hysterical symptoms. Firstly, the elements of this language were identified as iconic signs, and it was suggested that it be called protolanguage to set it apart from, and bring it into relation to, object and metalanguage. Secondly the relationship between the iconic signs of body language and the objects they denote was analysed. This type of inquiry is concerned with the cognitive uses of languages. Its purpose is to clarify the meaning of signs by elucidating the relationship between them and their referents (i.e. the objects to which they refer).

In the science of signs, concern with the cognitive uses of language is designated *semantics*. Semantics thus refers to the study of the relationship between signs and objects (or denotata). Truth and falsehood are semantical indices of the relationship between sign and object. Semantics must be contrasted with *pragmatics*, which adds the dimension of reference to persons. In pragmatics, one studies the three-fold relationship of sign–object–person. The statement 'This sentence is a law of physics' illustrates the pragmatic use of language (metalanguage), for it asserts that physicists consider the sentence true. Although the term 'semantics' has a more general, everyday meaning, designating all sorts of studies dealing with verbal communications, I shall use it here in its restricted sense.

Following Reichenbach's classification, we may distinguish three functions, or instrumental uses, of language: the informative, the affective, and the promotive.

The Informative Use of Protolanguage

The questions that arise here are: What kind of information is communicated by means of iconic body signs, and to whom? How effective is this mode of communication? What are its sources of error?

In order to answer these questions – that is, to identify the *pragmatics of protolanguage* – it is necessary to express our findings in ordinary language or in some logical refinement of it. Thus, we translate our initial observations or data into a symbol system other (and logically higher) than that in which they are first articulated.

The principal *informative* use of a typical hysterical body sign – once again, let us take as our example an hysterically paralysed arm – is to communicate to the recipient of the message that the sender is disabled. This may be phrased as: 'I am disabled', or 'I am sick', or 'I have been hurt', etc. The recipient for whom the message is intended may be an actual person or may be an internal object or parental image.

In everyday usage – and particularly in medical practice – the pragmatic use of body language is invariably *confused* with its cognitive use. In other words, when we translate the non-verbal communication of a non-functioning arm into the form 'I am sick' or 'My body is disordered', we equate and confuse a non-specific request for help with a request for a specific – in this case, *medical* – type of assistance. But in so far as the patient's statement is promotive, it should be translated as 'Do *something* for me!'

Although a purely cognitive analysis of such messages may be irrelevant and misleading, when physicians perform a differential diagnosis for an hysterical symptom, they address themselves to body signs as if they constituted cognitive communications. As a result, they come up with the answer 'Yes or No', or 'True or False'. But to say to a patient with a so-called conversion symptom, 'Yes, you are ill' – which is what Breuer and Freud did; or 'No, you are not ill (you malinger)' – which is what 'hardboiled' physicians tend to do, are both *incorrect*. This is because only semantically can an utterance be said to be true or false. Pragmatically, the issue is whether or not the recipient of the message believes what he has been told. Hence it is that, in so far as psychiatry is concerned with the study of sign-users, a purely semantic analysis of communications must necessarily fail to take account of some of the most significant aspects of the phenomena studied.

From the standpoint of pragmatic analysis, then, the traditional malingering approach to hysteria is essentially one of disbelief and rejection of the cognitive use of this type of communication. Conversely, the psychoanalytic attitude is characterized by the listener's belief in what the patient says; however, the belief is based on accepting the utterance only as a report and not as a true proposition. It is as if the analyst said to the patient: 'Yes, I believe that you believe that you are sick (meaning that your body is disordered). Your belief, however, is probably false. Indeed, you probably believe that you are sick – and want me to believe it – so that we should not have to deal with your "real troubles".' But usually none of this is *actually* said. And so both patient and analyst come to believe that the patient is somehow truly sick – though just how remains inexplicit.

If we want to distinguish among various types of communicational situations, we must ask whether a particular mode of communication serves to inform or whether it serves some other goal. The purpose of making small-talk is to participate in an easygoing, pleasant human relationship. The imparting of communicatively significant messages is not a necessary part of this situation. This may be contrasted with a teaching situation, in which the instructor must convey a certain amount of novel information to the students.

The same distinction must be made with respect to medicine and psychiatry. Each of these disciplines takes a different interest in and attitude towards body signs. Physicians, concerned with the functioning and breakdown of the human body as a machine, are committed to viewing body language as if it spoke in terms of cognitively significant messages. For instance, oppressive chest pain radiating into the left shoulder and arm in a middle-aged man is viewed as a message informing the physician of a coronary occlusion.

Psychoanalysts, on the other hand, are committed – not in the sense of an unalterable belief, but in the sense that this position is their characteristic operational attitude – to regarding bodily signs as cognitively insignificant, at least in the form in which they are presented. Thus, while the task of the physician is to diagnose and treat, the task of the psychoanalyst is to foster the self-reflective attitude in the patient towards his own body signs in order to facilitate their translation into verbal symbols. This process of translation, although it can be described in one simple sentence, is in practice a most difficult task. It constitutes, in my opinion, the core of what has been so misleadingly labelled the process of 'psychoanalytic treatment' or 'cure'.

The Affective Use of Protolanguage

The second function to which language may be put is deliberately to arouse certain emotions in the listener and so induce him to undertake certain actions. Reichenbach called this the suggestive, and I shall designate it as the affective, use of language. Poetry and propaganda, for example, typically serve this function. Few utterances are entirely free of an affective and promotive component.

The significance of the affective use of body language – or generally, of the language of illness – can hardly be exaggerated. The impact of hysterical pantomime, to use Freud's felicitous metaphor, is a matter of everyday knowledge. It is part of our social ethic – that is, of the rules by which we play the game of life – that we ought to feel sorry for sick people, and should try to be helpful to them. Communications by means of body signs may therefore be intended mainly to induce the following sort of feelings in the recipient: 'Aren't you sorry for me now?' 'You should be ashamed of yourself for having hurt me so!' 'You should be sad seeing how I suffer . . .' and so forth.

There are, of course, many other situations in which communications are used for a similar purpose. Among these are the ceremonial occasions during which the image of the crucified Christ is displayed. This spectacle affects the spectator as a mood-inducer, commanding him to feel humble, guilty, over-awed, and in general mentally constricted – and hence receptive to the messages of those who claim to speak for the man and the deed of which the statuette is an iconic sign. Similarly, *la grande hystérie* seen at the Salpêtrière, or the flamboyant 'schizophrenic bodily feelings' encountered today, represent communications in the contexts of specific social situations. Their aim is to suggest and induce mood rather than to convey cognitive information. And, in fact, they do induce mood as if the message had read: 'Pay attention to me!' 'Be impressed by how sick I am! (For I am outstanding at least in the horror and hopelessness of my illness.)' 'Be angry with me, and punish me, for look how angry and annoying I can be!' It is common knowledge that body language is very effective for inducing these and similar moods: for example, by shedding a few tears women can make most men do almost anything.

In general, whenever people feel unable to prevail by means of ordinary speech over the significant persons in their environment, they are likely to shift their pleas to the idiom of proto-language (e.g., weeping, body signs). When, in other words, one's love object fails to listen and respond to verbal complaints or requests, one will be compelled, or at least tempted, to take recourse in communicating by means of iconic body signs.[4] *We have come to speak of this general phenomenon, which may take a great variety of forms, as 'mental illness'.* As a result, instead of realizing that people are engaged in various types of communications in diverse communicational (or social) situations, we construct – and then ourselves come to believe in – various types of mental illnesses, such as 'hysteria', 'hypochondriasis', 'schizophrenia', and so forth.

The Promotive Use of Protolanguage

The third function of language, the promotive, is to make the listener perform certain actions. Commands such as 'Thou shalt not steal' or 'Turn right' illustrate this usage. Employing the imperative form makes the promotive use of language explicit. However, indicative sentences may also be used promotively, as for example, in the sentence 'All men are created equal.' Although ostensibly a descriptive assertion, it is clear that the statement was intended to be, and can only be, prescriptive and promotive.

Prescriptive assertions cannot be labelled either 'true' or 'false'. Reichenbach (1947) suggested a simple method for transforming pragmatical relations into statements that may be said to be 'true' or 'false' – namely, by making statements explicitly including the sign-user:

Thus to the imperative 'shut the door' we can co-ordinate the indicative sentence 'Mr A. wishes the door to be shut.' This sentence is true or false. (p. 19)

[4] These observations suggest that the informative use of language is most effective in egalitarian or 'free' situations. In this type of situation, information will, as a rule, induce the asked-for action. Or it will evoke some sort of counter-information. On the other hand, when a powerless person seeks aid from a relatively more powerful one, he must usually resort to the affective use of language. Simply asking for something would only expose his own weakness. In contrast, the exhibition of violent suffering might, by making the other party anxious and guilty, bring about the desired action.

The indicative sentence, however, may not have the instrumental (promotive) function which the prescriptive sentence had.

The masquerading of promotive assertions in the guise of indicative sentences is of great practical significance in psychiatry. Statements concerning 'psychosis' or 'insanity', involving persons other than the psychiatrist and the patient, almost always revolve around unclarified equations of these two linguistic forms. For example, the statement 'John Doe is psychotic' is ostensibly indicative and informative. Usually, however, it is promotive rather than informative, and may be translated – by explicitly including the sign-users – as follows: Mrs John Doe does not like the way her husband is acting. Dr James Smith believes that men preoccupied by jealousy are 'crazy' and potentially dangerous. Hence, both Mrs Doe and Dr Smith want Mr Doe to be confined in a hospital. Clearly, however, the indicative sentences do not have nearly the same promotive impact as does the much shorter assertion that 'John Doe is psychotic.'

If language is used promotively and expresses neither truth nor falsehood, what does one say in response to it? The answer is that one promotive usage must be opposed by another. Words like 'right' and 'wrong', which are themselves imperatives, perform this function. The command 'Thou shalt not steal' may thus be countered by saying either 'right' or 'wrong', depending on whether we agree or disagree with this rule.

The most obvious function of body language is its promotive use. By communicating through such 'symptoms' as headache, backache, or menstrual pains a housewife who feels over-burdened or dissatisfied with her life may be able to make her husband more attentive and helpful. And if not her husband, then perhaps her physician. And if not her physician, then perhaps some specialist to whom he might refer her. And so forth. This action-inducing meaning of iconic body signs may be paraphrased as follows: ('I am sick, therefore . . .) Take care of me!' – 'Be good to me!' – 'Make my husband do such and such!' – 'Tell my draft board to stop bothering me!' – 'Tell the court and the judge that I was not responsible!' And so forth.

From the viewpoint of our present analysis, the entire change in renaming certain illnesslike forms of behaviour from 'malingering' to 'hysteria' (and 'mental illness') can be understood as nothing but a linguistic change employed for the purpose of achieving a new type of action-orientation. This verbal change, as first advocated by Charcot, served to command those charged with dealing with 'hysterics' to abandon their rejecting attitude towards them and to adopt instead a benevolent attitude, such as befitted a physician vis-à-vis his patient.

7 Hysteria as Communication

Hysteria as Non-discursive Language

Logic, mathematics, and the sciences employ language only, or predominantly, to transmit information. Indeed, probably because science is so intimately associated with the informative use of language, scientists and philosophers have repeatedly suggested that 'the essential business of language is to assert or deny facts' (Russell, 1922, p. 8). This is true, however, only for the language of science, mathematics, and logic, and is false for sign-using behaviour encountered in many other situations. As Rapoport (1954) aptly observed:

It is not necessary to look into books on philosophy to find words without referents. Any commencement speech, sermon, newspaper editorial, or radio commercial follows the same philosophic tradition of reinforcing the delusion that anything which is talked about is real: success, charity, public opinion, and four-way indigestion relief. Indeed, nothing is easier than to 'define' these noises so as to make it appear that they mean something. (p. 18)

These 'noises' of everyday speech, which have a great deal in common with the 'noises' of psychiatric symptoms, require that we consider the second principal function of language, namely, the expression of emotions, feelings, or desires. These expressions are, according to most modern students of language, not symbols for thought but symptoms of the inner life of the speaker. In *Philosophy in a New Key* (1942), Langer criticized this view and suggested that there was a necessity for a 'genuine semantic beyond the limits of discursive language' (p. 70). Although Langer made some tentative suggestions about the directions in which this semantic might be sought, particularly with respect to music and the visual arts, her work in this regard remained programmatic. One of my aims in this book is to implement this programme by providing a *systematic semiotical analysis of a language-form hitherto regarded as purely expressive, i.e. the language of certain bodily signs.*

Discursive and Non-discursive Languages

In addition to classifying languages according to their logical complexity, they may also be classified according to the degree of their discursiveness. *Discursiveness is a measure of the degree of arbitrariness of symbolization.* Mathematics and the languages of the various sciences serve the sole function of transmitting information. Non-discursive – or, more precisely, relatively slightly discursive – languages, on the other hand, serve mainly the purpose of emotional expression. Art, dance, and the ritual are characteristic examples. In these communications, symbolization is *idiosyncratic* rather than *conventional*.

In this connection Langer emphasized the special significance of the picture as symbol, noting that the photograph of a person does not describe the man who posed for it but rather presents a replica of him (pp. 76–7). For this reason, non-discursive symbolism is often called *presentational*. It is evident, too, that while discursive symbolism has primarily a general reference, a presentational symbol refers to a specific, individual object. The former is thus eminently *abstract*, the latter exquisitely *concrete*. The word 'man' refers to every conceivable man – and even woman! – in the universe, but points to no specific person. The photograph of a man, on the other hand, represents and identifies a particular person.

In the earliest forms of written language, formal representation was achieved by means of iconic signs – that is, by hieroglyphs, which constitute a form of picture writing. According to Schlauch (1942), the two simplest elements in written language are pictographs and ideographs. Both express their messages by means of pictures that *resemble* the object or idea to be conveyed. They could be regarded as the earliest prototypes of what we now call the analogic type of codification. *Kinesics* (Birdwhistell, 1949) could thus be said to be a modern attempt to explore and understand *the hieroglyphics that a person writes, not on marble tablets, but on and with his own body.*

The advantages of discursive symbolism for transmitting information are known and generally appreciated. The question that now arises is whether non-discursive symbolism has any function besides that of expressing emotions? Indeed, it has several such functions.

Since verbal symbols *describe* the objects they denote in a relatively general, abstract fashion, the identification of a specific object requires much circumlocution (unless it has a *name*, which is a very special kind of discursive sign).

For this reason [wrote Langer (1942)] the correspondence between a word-picture and a visible object can never be as close as that between the object and its photograph. Given all at once to the intelligent eye, an incredible wealth and detail of information is conveyed by the portrait, where we do not have to stop to construe verbal meanings. That is why we use a photograph rather than a description on a passport or in the Rogues' Gallery. (p. 77)

It is evident, then, that so-called hysterical body signs, *as pictures,* bear a much greater similarity to the objects which they depict than do words describing the same objects.[1] To exhibit, by means of bodily signs – say, by paralyses or convulsions – the idea and message that one is sick is at once more striking and more informative than simply saying: 'I am sick.' *Body signs portray – they literally present and represent – in exactly what way the sufferer considers himself sick.* Thus, in the symbolism of his symptom, the patient could be said to present his own complaint and – albeit in a highly condensed form – even his autobiography. This is tacitly recognized by psychoanalysts who often treat the patient's presenting symptom – if he has one – as if it contained the whole history and structure of his 'neurosis'. When psychoanalysts say that even the simplest symptom can be understood fully only in retrospect, they mean

[1] Treating certain forms of behaviour as pictures, used to communicate messages, also helps us to comprehend such everyday acts as wearing certain distinctive articles of clothing (e.g. caps, jackets, the use of pipes, etc.). Such 'dressing up' behaviour is like saying: 'I belong to this group', or 'I am so and so' (as a means of self-identification, e.g. 'I am a Harvard man'). Uniforms, of course, are used deliberately to bestow a specific identity or role on a person, such as 'You are in the navy, now', or 'You are an officer', etc. In all these situations we deal with the social uses of iconic signs.

that in order to understand the patient's 'symptom' we must be acquainted with all the historically unique aspects of his personality development and social circumstances.

The situation in regard to cases of typical organic disease is quite different. The patient's symptom – say, angina pectoris (due to coronary insufficiency) – is not autobiographical; in other words, it is not personal and idiosyncratic, at least not characteristically so. Instead, the symptom is anatomically and physiologically determined. The structure of the body defines, within limits, its function. Substernal pain cannot be the sign of, say, a ruptured ovarian cyst. Knowledge of pathological anatomy and physiology thus makes it possible to infer the 'meaning' of the 'messages' of certain bodily symptoms. To make similar inferences from iconic symbolism, however, it is of no use to be familiar with the language of medicine. What is needed, instead, is familiarity with the personality of the sign-user, including his family background, personal history, religion, occupation, and so forth. Accordingly, although so-called psychiatric symptoms are idiosyncratic (in the sense that they are personal), they may be shown to exhibit certain patterns of regularity. These will depend on the patient's personal and social experiences – in brief, on what he has learned as a human being. The experienced or intuitive psychotherapist is one who is familiar with the 'meanings' of the predominant patterns of 'psychiatric symptoms' or difficulties in a given culture or situation.

It is to be expected, then, that the non-discursive or presentational form of symbolism should readily lend itself to the expression and communication of so-called psychiatric problems. Such problems pertain to personal difficulties that are, by nature, concrete experiences. Human beings have troubles with their mothers, fathers, brothers, and so forth as *individuals* – as *concrete human beings*. They do not suffer from the effects of Oedipal complexes or sexual instincts as abstractions. It follows, then, that iconic body signs have the advantage of fitting specifically the objects to which they refer. Such signs and most 'psychiatric symptoms' do not, like the symbols of ordinary language, have a general reference, but point rather to specific individuals or events. The transformation (for it cannot properly be called translation) of presentational symbols into conventional signs (ordinary words), such as occurs in the course of psycho-analysis and some forms of psychotherapy, must thus be seen as itself constituting a process of personality change. This does not necessarily mean that verbalization is the most significant feature of psychological 'treatment'. Nor should this idea be confused with the early psychoanalytic notion of 'catharsis'. On the contrary, a semiotical analysis of psychiatric operations should enable us to see more clearly, and to describe more accurately, the precise mechanisms by which talking often helps people to cope with their problems in living.

The Non-discursiveness of Hysteria

To illustrate that the communicative aspects of hysterical symptoms are incomprehensible in terms of the logic of everyday speech, let us consider some of Freud's clinical observations, cited earlier. Remarking on the differences between organic and hysterical pains, Freud (Breuer and Freud, 1893–5) wrote:

I was struck by the indefiniteness of all the descriptions of the character of her pains given me by the patient, who was nevertheless a highly intelligent person. A patient suffering from *organic pains* will, unless he is *neurotic in addition*, describe them *definitely and calmly*. He will say, for instance, that they are shooting pains, that they occur at certain intervals, that they seem to him to be brought on by one thing or another. Again, when a *neurasthenic describes his pains*, he gives an impression of being engaged in a difficult intellectual task to which his strength is quite unequal. He is clearly of the opinion that *language is too poor to find words for his sensations* and that these sensations are something unique and previously unknown, of which it would be quite impossible to give an exhaustive description. ([Italics added] p. 136)

Freud's account shows how exceedingly difficult it is for the patient to find words for his so-called sensations. The same holds true for patients expressing bodily feelings associated with psychiatric syndromes other than hysteria (e.g. hypochondriasis, schizophrenia, depression). This phenomenon has been generally explained by assuming that the patient has unusual or peculiar feelings, difficult to put into words; or by attributing it to a general impoverishment in the patient's use of verbal language.

Let me suggest still another explanation. The symptom – say, a pain or bodily feeling – may be part of a symbol system, albeit not of a discursive type. The difficulty in expressing the 'feeling' in verbal language is due to the fact that non-discursive languages do not lend themselves to translation into other idioms, least of all into discursive forms. The referents of non-discursive symbols have meaning only if the communicants are attuned to each other. This is in harmony with the actual operations of psychoanalysis: analytic technique rests on the tacit assumption that we cannot know – in fact, must not even expect to know – what troubles our patients until we have become attuned to them.

The Informative Function of Iconic Body Signs

To what extent, or precisely how, can non-discursive languages be used to transmit information? This question has occupied philosophers and students of signs for some time. More particularly, the informative function of a special type of non-discursive language, namely, of so-called hysterical body signs, has long been of interest to psychiatrists. Although hysteria has been approached *as if it were a language*, it has never been systematically so codified. Let us therefore consider the *informative uses of iconic body signs as a system of non-discursive language*.[2]

In general, the informative use of language depends on the referents of its symbols. The radical positivist view, probably rarely held today, maintains that non-discursive languages have no referents at all: messages framed in this idiom are held to be meaningless. A more balanced and, I think, today more widely accepted philosophical position regards the difference between discursive and non-discursive languages as a matter of degree rather than kind. Hence, non-discursive languages, too, have referents and cognitive meaning.

Rapoport (1954), for example, suggested that the referents of

[2] This analysis will apply to phenomena variously labelled 'hysteria', 'hypochondriasis', 'schizophrenia', and so forth. The distinguishing feature is the use of *body signs* and their *iconicity*. The labels of traditional psychiatric nosology are of no use in ascertaining where or when we may encounter such signs.

non-discursive symbols are the 'inner states' of the communicants. Although Rapoport recognized that non-discursive languages have referents, he nevertheless adhered to a traditional 'out there – in here' distinction between them. He thus regarded discursive referents as ideally suited for conveying information, and non-discursive referents as having the function of transmitting a feeling state from one person to another. The latter is a familiar phenomenon in clinical psychiatry, and also in the arts.

It is true, of course, that non-discursive communication is simple and concrete. Still, it is *not merely* a communication of the sender's inner experience. Let us consider, in this connection, the example of people fleeing a burning theatre. The panicky behaviour of some members of the audience may signify – even to someone who neither sees flames nor hears anyone shout 'Fire!' – *more* than mere panic. At first, perhaps, one may respond to the purely affective function of body language: 'People around me are afraid, panicky: I, too, *feel* panicky.' Yet, closely connected with this, there is a communication of a quasi-cognitive message: 'I am in danger! I must flee to save myself, or otherwise make sure that I shall be safe (e.g. by checking whether a danger really threatens).'

I cite this case to show that the referent *inside* a communicant – say, his affect – cannot be completely severed from the experiencing person's *relationship to the world about him*. This is because affects are at once private – 'inner referents', and public – indices of relationships between ego and object(s), self and others (Szasz, 1957a). Affects are thus the primary link between inner, private experiences – and outer, publicly verifiable, occurrences. Herein lies the ground for assigning more than only subjective, idiosyncratic meanings to the referents of non-discursive languages. Accordingly, the limitation of iconic body signs does not lie solely in the subjectiveness of the experience and its expression – that is, in the fact that no one can feel another's pain; it lies, rather, in the fact that such signs present a picture – say, of a person writhing in pain – which, standing alone, has a very limited cognitive content.

The study of *gestures* is pertinent in this connection. Gesture is the earliest faculty of communication, the 'elder brother of speech' (Critchley, p. 121). This developmental fact is consistent with the relatively primitive cognitive use to which this form of communication may be put, and with the equally primitive learning (imitation, identification) which it subserves. In semiotical terms, gesture is a highly iconic system of signs, verbal speech is only very slightly iconic, while mathematics is completely non-iconic.

Concrete, action-oriented gestures are manifestations of an early stage in the maturational history of the human being as a *social animal*. The ability to wait, to defer action, to inhibit impulses, are aspects of psychosocial maturation. Together, as they are displayed in the increasingly complex uses of symbols, they constitute the differences between child and adult.

Hysteria, Translation, and Misinformation

When hysterical body signs are used to transmit information, they exhibit the same limitations as do non-discursive languages generally. Weakly discursive languages cannot be readily translated into more strongly discursive ones. When such translation is attempted, the possibilities for error are enormous, since virtually *any* discursive rendition of the original message will, in a sense, be false! There are two basic reasons, then, why hysterical symptoms so often *misinform*: one is the linguistic difficulty, just noted, of rendering non-discursive symbolism into discursive form; the other is that the message may actually be intended for an internal object and not for the recipient who actually receives and interprets it.

Misinformation is bound to be generated whenever a communication framed in the idiom of iconic body signs is interpreted in the language of medicine. Typical is the case of the patient who 'says' that he is sick by means of hysterical pantomime, but whose communication the physician interprets by making a diagnosis. Since in the special scientific idiom of medicine 'sickness' means a disorder of the body, the patient's original message will necessarily be mistranslated.

Of course, misinformation – whether it be a mistake or a lie – may be communicated by means of ordinary language as well as by iconic body signs. We speak of a lie when the misinformation is considered to serve the speaker's interests and when it is believed that he has sent the false message deliberately. A mistake, by contrast, is an error made indifferently. Hence, there can be no such thing as a 'deliberate mistake', but mistakes out of ignorance or lack of skill (conditions which might themselves be the results of deliberate planning) can occur.

In describing this contrast between lying and making a mistake I have deliberately avoided the concept of consciousness. The traditional psychoanalytic idea that so-called conscious imitation of illness is 'malingering' and hence 'not illness', whereas its allegedly unconscious simulation is itself 'illness', that is, 'hysteria', creates more problems than it solves. I think it is more useful to *distinguish between goal-directed and rule-following behaviour on the one hand, and indifferent mistakes on the other*. In psychoanalytic theory there is no room for indifferent mistakes – because it is tacitly assumed that all action is goal-directed. It then follows that a person's failure to perform adequately cannot be due to his ignorance of the rules of the game or to his lack of skills in playing it. Instead, the failure itself is regarded as a goal, albeit an unconscious one. This perspective, and the therapeutic attitude it inspires, are exceedingly useful. Yet it is obvious that not all human error is of this purposive kind. To insist on this view is to deny the very possibility of genuine error.

By reintroducing the distinction between goal-directed misinformation and indifferent error into psychiatry and psychoanalysis, I believe we shall be able to clarify many problems in human behaviour. In the case of hysteria, for example, Freud himself emphasized the quasi-rational, goal-directed nature of the process. In short, *it is more accurate to regard hysteria as a lie than as a mistake*. People caught in a lie usually maintain that they were merely mistaken. The difference between mistakes and lies, when discovered, is chiefly pragmatic.[3] From a purely cognitive point of view, both are simply falsehoods.

[3] What is meant by this is that we hold people responsible for lies but not, as a rule, for mistakes. We touch here on the immense problem of the observer's *attitude* towards various forms of personal conduct: for it depends largely on how behaviour is *judged* whether it will be rewarded, ignored, punished, treated as illness, etc.

Language as a Means of Making Contact with Objects[4]

The study of hysteria, and of psychiatric problems generally, places Donne's famous utterance, 'No man is an island, entire of itself', in a new perspective. Human beings *need* other human beings. This need cannot be reduced to other, more elementary, needs. Freud himself went far in elucidating the young child's vast need for and hence dependence on his parents, especially his mother or mother substitute. Indeed, *regression* was one of Freud's key explanatory concepts. By this it was meant that, generally speaking, man finds psychosocial maturation burdensome. Thus, he has a tendency to return to earlier, psychosocially less complex modes of functioning. Implicit in this concept is the idea that when human contact at some later level proves unendurable, contact is sought at an earlier, more easily satisfied level.

The psychology of object relationships – the quintessence of present-day psychoanalysis – *presupposes* the need for objects. So viewed, *the task of psychoanalysis is to study and elucidate the kinds of objects people need, and the exact ways in which they need them.* Some generalizations may be formulated. For example, children have a greater need for supportive external objects than adults who often turn to internal objects for such help. A great deal of recent psychoanalytic literature is devoted to discussions of the various mechanisms for seeking and maintaining object relationships. Emphasis on an object-relationship point of view has made it possible to interpret such phenomena as touching, caressing, cuddling and, of course, sexual intercourse itself as a means of *making contact* with objects.

There is no reason to assume that what is true for gestural (non-verbal) communications is not also true for verbal language. Since all communicative behaviour is addressed to someone, it has, among other functions, also the aim of making contact with another human being. We may call this *the object-seeking and relationship-maintaining function of language*. The significance

[4] I use the term 'object' here in the psychoanalytic sense to refer to persons or to objects invested with personal qualities (e.g. dolls).

and success of this function varies with the discursiveness of the particular idiom. If the main aim of the communication is to establish human contact, the language used to achieve it will be relatively non-discursive (e.g. chitchat, small-talk, dancing, 'schizophrenic' bodily symptoms). Because of this, we are justified in treating relatively slightly discursive communications mainly as methods of making contact with people rather than as methods of communicating information.

This viewpoint lends special poignancy to the interpretation of such things as the dance, music, religious ritual, and the representative arts. In all of these, the participant or viewer can enter into a significant relationship with a person by means of the non-discursive sign system employed. Using a pharmaceutical analogy, it is as if the language – dance, art, etc. – were the vehicle in which the active ingredient – human contact – is suspended and contained. Many things that people do together have mainly this function, whether it be playing bridge or tennis, going hunting with a friend, or attending a scientific meeting. To be sure, these situations serve other purposes as well. The hunter, though sharing his experience with a friend, may have to feed his family. The person attending a scientific meeting may also learn something from the lectures. These instrumental tasks are, however, often overshadowed by the human relationship aspects of the situation.

Traditionally, language has been viewed as serving the purpose of transmitting information from one person to another, an assumption which has obscured its object-seeking and relationship-maintaining functions. Consider, for example, the biblical account of God speaking to Moses. Their communication was in *earnest*. They did not chat to satisfy their need for companionship. Instead, God gave Moses the *Law*. The Divine Law is regarded, of course, as a piece of suprahuman 'truth', or, in philosophical terms, the quintessence of the positivist's conception of a 'logical assertion'. But surely nowadays communications in a formally religious setting serve chiefly the function of seeking and maintaining object relationships. Hence, irrespective of what religious propositions might lack from a cognitive point of view, they satisfy the worshipper's needs for objects. Herein lies the main reason for the relative ineffectiveness of logical arguments and empirical demonstrations against religious, national, and professional myths.

The foregoing illustration also demonstrates the general intellectual tendency to assume that the important thing in verbal communication is the logical content of the message. We look for all sorts of meanings in language, and rightly so. This very meaningfulness, however, conceals the non-specific, object-seeking function of language. Hence, people are most apt to recognize this function only when the meaning of the communication is blatantly unimportant or absent, as in what we call 'chitchat'. But the object-seeking function of language is nearly always important. In the small child, it is manifested by incessant questions such as: 'Daddy, what is this, where does it come from, can we have some, can we do this?' Intelligence, curiosity, or the wish to explore the environment may all have something to do with this type of behaviour. But the child has also learned that the *exchange of verbal communications* is an effective and gratifying method for being with another person. In this sense, speaking and listening are displaced and sophisticated forms of seeing, touching, or cuddling. This is why a few words in the dark, or the parents' quiet conversation in another room, reassure the fearful child.

The object-seeking function of language is most important during the early years of life. With psychological maturation, its significance is replaced by the informative function of communication. This transformation is shown in condensed form in Table 4. The foremost aim of the child's earliest communications is often to seek objects and to maintain contact with them. As maturation progresses, this 'grasping' function of language diminishes. Gradually, situations of mutual interest arise: children learn to use language abstractly. Serious psychological commitment to reading and writing implies an orientation to persons not physically present. While verbal language, as well as the special languages of science, retain an object-seeking aspect, this becomes increasingly less personal.

Abstract symbol-systems, such as mathematics, are especially valuable for object-seeking for schizoid personalities. By means of such symbolizations object contact may be sought and obtained, while at the same time a psychological distance may

TABLE 4. DEVELOPMENT OF THE OBJECT-SEEKING FUNCTION OF LANGUAGE

Developmental Stage	Typical Communications and their Effects on the Recipient	Linguistic Characteristics	What Is Gained and/or Learned?
The baby's cry	Crying, weeping, bodily manifestations of suffering and discomfort: 'Feel like me!' 'Come to me!'	Non-verbal, non-discursive, high degree of iconicity	Early identifications; maintenance of the organism
The child's verbal complaint	'It hurts!' 'I can't sleep!' 'Take care of me!' 'Don't leave me!'	Verbal, non-discursive, reduced degree of iconicity	Internalization of objects and building of the self
The child's questioning	'What is it called?' 'Where does it come from?' 'Can we have some?'	Verbal, increasingly discursive, non-iconic (conventional) signs	Internalization of objects; acquisition of information or knowledge
The adolescent's intelligent conversation	Intellectual curiosity: 'Talk to me,' 'Be interested in me (my mind).' 'Respect me for my thoughts and knowledge.'	Verbal, increasingly discursive	Same as above; identification as adult by relating to adult objects; increasing emphasis on knowledge as a source of self-esteem
The (young) adult student's communicative attitude towards his teacher	The wish for personal instruction: 'Teach me!'	Verbal or special discursive symbol systems	Symbols, skills, and knowledge. (Gradually diminishing interest in teacher as person.)
Communication with books	The wish to learn impersonally: 'Teach me!' as a message addressed to a physically absent person	Same as above	Same as above in a context of individual achievement
Communication with others in a co-operative situation	The wish to learn in a co-operative enterprise; not 'Teach me!' but rather 'We shall participate together, exchange ideas and skills, and learn from each other.'	Same as above	Same as above in a context of co-operative achievement

be maintained between self and other; it is virtually impossible to have a personal relationship and at the same time maintain such distance. The fascination with and value of abstractions – whether as 'addiction' to books or as religious or scientific systems – lie precisely in this. Yet, for persons employing such schizoid strategies, the lack of concreteness of the object and the ego's persistent lack of contact with actual people contribute further to an already troublesome alienation from the world of human beings and hence remain a constant source of danger for them.

. The object-seeking function of hysteria is especially significant for the work of psychotherapy. Freud's essential thesis was that hysteria constituted a behavioural technique invoked by patients, especially women, when they could reach their love-object in no other way. When verbal communications, such as pleading and explanations failed, they resorted to hysteria in the hope that it might succeed. Thus, a woman unable to enlist her husband's sympathy, attention, and interest under so-called normal circumstances, succeeded in doing so when she 'fell ill with hysteria'. This important social fact has as much to do with the psychology of the receiver of messages as with that of the sender. Certain non-verbal communications – such as crying or temper tantrums – make a much greater impact on the receiver than do communications framed in the idiom of polite conversation. While the latter can be ignored, the former cannot. Hysterical pantomime, much like the demands of children, exerts a powerful effect on the person to whom it is directed. Confronted with so-called hysterical symptoms, therapists as well as marriage partners find it extremely difficult *not* to *respond*. And since what is sought is, at least partly, a response – *any* response, as it indicates interest and affection – *the value* of hysteria (and of many other so-called mental illnesses) as a method for making contact with an object is very real indeed. This, however, must not be confused either with 'primary' or 'secondary gain'. The object-seeking value of iconic body signs contains elements of both primary and secondary gain, in that both of these refer to ends which themselves presuppose relationship with an object.

Hysteria as Indirect Communication

Highly discursive languages, such as mathematics, permit only direct communications. Mathematical signs have clearly defined referents, accepted by the mutual agreement of all who engage in 'conversation' in this idiom. Ambiguity and misunderstanding are thus reduced to a minimum.

The principal linguistic cause of misunderstanding is ambiguity. In ordinary language many signs are employed in several different senses, a circumstance that allows for much ambiguity and hence misunderstanding. At the same time, referential ambiguity allows one to make indirect communications intentionally, by employing expressions known to be interpretable in more than one way. It is precisely that some types of communications have *multiple meanings* that make them suitable as methods of indirect communication.

The difference between indirectness and non-discursiveness may now be stated. A language is called non-discursive not because its signs have a multiplicity of well-defined referents, but rather because the referents are idiosyncratic and, hence, *poorly* defined. Directness and discursiveness overlap at one end, in that highly discursive expressions are also direct. They do not overlap at the other end, for non-discursiveness itself is no guarantee that the language is useful for indirect communications. For this purpose a language of some discursiveness, such as ordinary language, is more useful than one that is completely non-discursive, such as music.

There are many terms for various kinds of indirect communications – such as hinting, alluding, speaking in metaphor, double talk, insinuation, implication, punning, and so forth. Significantly, while hinting is neutral in regard to what is being alluded to, insinuation refers only to depreciatory allusions. Moreover, insinuation has no antonym: there is no expression to describe insinuating something 'good' about someone. Although flattery might at times be communicated by allusion, the fact that no special word exists for it provides linguistic support for the thesis that hinting serves mainly to protect a speaker who is afraid to offend.

The Psychology of Hinting

Whenever language is used to transmit information, direct communications will predominate. So-called statements of facts, logical propositions, and scientific discourse generally, consist of direct communications. Their aim is to communicate by means of maximally concise and unambiguous messages. The affectional relationship between the communicants – that is, whether or not they like each other – is, in these circumstances, quite irrelevant.

On the other hand, when the relationship between two people is emotionally significant but uncertain – or when either feels dependent or threatened or inhibited by the other – then the stage is set for the exchange of indirect messages between them. There is good reason for this – namely, that indirect messages serve two useful functions – firstly, to transmit information, and secondly, to *explore and modify the relationship* between the communicants. This exploratory function of indirect communications may include the aim of attempting, however subtly, to change the other person's attitude to make him more receptive to our needs and desires.

Dating and courtship provide many excellent illustrations of indirect communications. In dating, for example, the boy may want uncomplicated sex play and perhaps sexual intercourse. The girl may or may not share this interest. In the initial stages of the dating game neither knows how the other wants to play. Often they do not even know precisely what game they are going to play. Moreover, in our culture direct communications about sexual interests and activities are discouraged, even prohibited. Hinting and alluding thus become indispensable methods of communication.

Indirect messages permit communicative contacts when, without them, the alternatives would be total inhibition, silence, and solitude on the one hand, or, on the other, communicative behaviour that is direct, offensive, and hence forbidden. These alternatives are painful. In actual practice, neither is likely to result in the gratification of the needs motivating the behaviour. In this dilemma, indirect communications provide a useful compromise. As one of the early moves in the dating game, the boy might invite the girl to dinner or to the cinema. These communications are polyvalent: the boy's suggestion and the girl's response to it have several 'levels' of meaning. One is the level of the overt message – that is, whether they will have dinner together, go to a movie, and so forth. Another, more covert, level pertains to the question of sexual activity: acceptance of the dinner invitation implies that sexual overtures might perhaps follow. Conversely, rejection of the invitation means not only refusal of companionship for dinner but also of the possibility of further sexual exploration. There may be still other levels of meaning. For instance, acceptance of the offer may be interpreted as a sign of personal (sexual) worth and hence ground for increased self-esteem, whereas rejection may mean the opposite and generate feelings of worthlessness.

Freud was a master at elucidating the psychological function of indirect communications. Speaking of the patient's associations to neurotic symptoms, he wrote: 'The idea occurring to the patient must be in the nature of an *allusion* to the repressed element, like a representation of it in indirect speech' (Freud, 1910a, p. 30). The concept of indirect communication occupies a central position in Freud's theory of dream work and neurotic symptom formation. He compared dream formation to the difficulty which confronts 'the political writer who has disagreeable truths to tell those in authority' (Freud, 1900, p. 141). The political writer, like the dreamer, cannot speak directly. The censor will not allow it. Hence, each must avail himself of 'indirect representations' (pp. 141–2).

Metaphorical communication is also a frequent source of jokes, cartoons, and humour of all sorts. Why is the story of the rich playboy asking the aspiring actress to come to his apartment to view his etchings funny? It is evident that the man is not interested in showing his etchings, nor the woman in looking at them, but that both are interested in sex. The man is interested because it will give him pleasure, the woman perhaps because she will be rewarded in some material way. The same message conveyed in direct language – that is, telling of a man offering a woman, say, fifty dollars to go to bed with him – would be informative but not humorous.

Freud (1905c) attributed the pleasurable quality of humour to the saving of psychic energy. This explanation was based on a hypothetical energetic scheme according to which man is a self-contained psychological machine, designed to minimize energy output and maximize available or stored energy (libido). Yet it is apparent that Freud was well aware of the linguistic finesses involved in humour. He did not, however, offer a linguistic – or semiotical – analysis of humour, dreams, and various psychological 'symptoms'.[5]

A semiotical analysis of humour has much in common with modern psychoanalytic ego-psychological interpretations of this phenomenon. Both attribute the pleasurable affects of humour to the successful mastery of a communicative task. For instance, in the girl-being-asked-to-see-an-etching situation, the scene is humorous only if the message is simultaneously interpreted in more than one way. If a metaphor, proverb, or joke is taken literally – as such linguistic forms often are by children, the unsophisticated, persons who do not speak the language well, or so-called schizophrenics – they are neither funny nor interesting. Their psychologically rewarding character derives entirely from the challenge and successful mastery of an ambiguous or polyvalent message.

The Protective Function of Indirect Communications

The protective function of hinting is especially important when communications are motivated by ego-alien or socially alien wishes, or by needs that are not apt to be satisfied. In our culture, therefore, indirect messages are often used to communicate sexual and dependency needs and problems about money. Faced with such 'delicate' matters, indirect communications permit the expression of a need and its simultaneous

[5] From an operational point of view, much of psychoanalysis revolves around the analysis of language. That psychoanalysis is, in a sense, a study of communications has been accepted as a matter of course by many analysts. These considerations notwithstanding, it must be emphasized that Freud's work was cast in the framework of medicine and psychiatry (medical psychology). The terms 'neurosis', 'psychosis', 'neurotic symptoms', 'psychoanalytic treatment' – to name but a few – are eloquent testimony to the medical heritage Freud acquired and from which he freed himself only to a very limited extent.

denial or disavowal. A classic example from medical practice is the physician's reluctance to discuss fees with patients and to handle money – tasks usually entrusted to a secretary or nurse. The physician communicating through his employee is simultaneously asking for money *and* not asking for money. The first message is contained *explicitly* in the secretary's request; the second is contained *implicitly* in the doctor's avoidance of the subject. Since the secretary is acting as the physician's agent, in a practical sense the physician is asking for money. From a psychological point of view, however, by not discussing financial matters, the physician is in effect saying that money is of no importance in his relationship with the patient. Much of what is called hypocrisy may thus be understood as indirect communication, serving, as a rule, the interests of the speaker and infringing correspondingly on the interests of the listener.

In the example cited, the indirect communication permits the physician to enhance his self-esteem by claiming that he is 'above' certain basic human needs (in this case, the need for money and all that it may buy and imply). This phenomenon derives from the premise, widely held in our culture, that the existence and open expression of needs is a childish characteristic, undesirable for 'normal' or socially admirable human relationships. The basis for this notion – a detailed consideration of which is beyond the scope of this presentation – is probably partly the fact that children possess large needs and little ability to regulate and satisfy them, and partly that the socialization of the child aims towards teaching him to deny, alter, regulate, and otherwise modify his needs. At the same time, the child is expected to become increasingly more self-reliant rather than dependent. Adults have thus convinced themselves that they are 'independent'. However, although adults may differ greatly from children, they can hardly be said to be independent. They too possess needs for whose satisfaction they require other people – including, still, the need for human contact. The differences between children and grown-ups lie mainly in the nature of their needs and their respective methods for satisfying them. The illusion of independence – one of man's self-aggrandizements – is thus supported by the use of indirect communications.

Whether a person considers bodily diseases and personal problems acceptable or unacceptable will depend on his system of values. In today's health-conscious atmosphere, bodily diseases are acceptable, but problems in living – lip-service to the contrary notwithstanding – are not. Indeed, they are *especially unacceptable in a medical setting*. Hence, people – patients and physicians alike – are inclined to deny personal problems and to communicate in terms of bodily illnesses: for example, a man worried about his job or marriage may seek medical attention for hyperacidity and insomnia; and his physician is likely to treat him with antacids and tranquillizers.

Hinting As Insurance Against Disappointment

How do indirect communications provide insurance against disappointment and object loss?

Let us take the example of a person in dire need of money. A direct request by begging can evoke only one of two responses. The request is either granted or rejected. This is because the message 'Please give me money!' is clear and cannot be mis-understood. Its disadvantage is that it leaves the speaker open to the rejection of his demand. Obviously, if direct repudiation of a request is feared, the forthright expression of wishes or needs will be inhibited. Indirect communication then becomes useful. For instance, in Central Europe between the two World Wars, many veterans, some of them disabled, were utterly destitute. They were forced to become beggars. However, they did not actually beg, but instead stood at street corners in their faded uniforms, silently offering something – a few pencils or outdated magazines – for sale. Similarly, in the United States during the early 1930s, unemployed men stood at street corners 'selling' apples.

In these examples, indirectness of communication is achieved by the fact that the needy person does not verbally request money or assistance. Ostensibly, he proclaims that he is selling something; actually, however, these 'vendors' sold things no-body wanted. If someone had wanted a pencil or an apple, he could have purchased it in the appropriate store. Moreover, the veterans would accept money without necessarily exchanging

147

merchandise for it. Viewing these situations in their totality, it is apparent that the 'beggar' or 'street vendor' was offering an indirect communication having the following structure:

1. Overtly, he was selling pencils or apples.

2. Covertly, he was begging.

3. As a veteran, displaying his uniform and perhaps also injuries and mutilations, he communicated – at once overtly and covertly – the wish to arouse sympathy and guilt in the passers-by. The injured veteran role implies that (*a*) as a vendor he was to be favoured over other vendors without his patriotic qualification, and (*b*) he was not to be identified with other non-veteran beggars.

The communicational *functions* of this situation were as follows:

1. The indigent person was enabled to *deny* or *obscure* the full magnitude of his unhappy socio-economic condition.

2. He could ask and be refused without the rejection being overtly codified. Hence, his pride and self-esteem were protected from further injury. This consideration can hardly be over-emphasized for someone whose self-image has already sustained a devastating blow. It might seem that such deception of one's self and others would hardly be necessary. But necessary it was, just as similar self-deceptions continue to be widely practised. The point to remember is that the more injured and vulnerable a person's self-image is, the greater will be his need to protect and bolster it. The observer's common-sense appraisal that self-protection by means of hinting is unnecessary is meaningless. What is necessary depends entirely on the experiencing person's perception of himself and the world about him.

3. Last but not least, the *communicational effectiveness* or *promotive power* of the indirect message was far greater than that of undisguised begging would have been. This was because begging was something shameful, while working and 'sacrificing for one's country' was something to be proud of. Moreover, a poor man asking for money directly, without offering work or merchandise in return for it, is regarded as aggressive. An indirect demand is experienced as more modest, and hence does not generate the angry resistance and rejection which an overt demand often does.

Keeping in mind the basic structure of this begging-vendorship situation, let us compare it with malingering and hysteria. Malingering, as I suggested, may be regarded as a type of impersonation: a man who is not sick acts as if he were. The same holds for indirect communications. In the example cited, a man who was not a vendor acted *as if* he had been one. In the first case, being ill or the *sick role* is impersonated; in the second, selling or the *vendor role* is.

In short, so long as we are willing to care for and protect those who are sick or disabled, impersonating the sick role will be useful to some people in certain circumstances. Hence, it is logically absurd to expect that hysteria could be eradicated as if it were a disease like malaria or smallpox.

Dreaming and Hysteria as Hinting

The main advantage of hinting over more direct modes of communication is the protection it affords the speaker by enabling him to communicate without committing himself to what he says. Should the message be ill received, hinting leaves an escape route open. Indirect communications ensure the speaker that he will be held responsible only for the explicit meaning of his message. The overt message thus serves as an envelope within which is contained the dangerous, hidden message – the covert communication.

Dreaming As Hinting

Any reported dream may be regarded as an indirect communication or a hint. The manifest dream story is the ostensible, overt message, while the latent dream thoughts constitute the covert message to which the dreamer alludes. This function of dreaming – and of dream-communication – is best observed in the psychoanalytic situation, since in it the recounting of dreams is a fully acceptable form of social behaviour. Analytic patients often produce dreams that refer to the analyst. Frequently, such dreams reveal that the analysand has some feeling or knowledge about the analyst which he finds distressing and is afraid to mention lest the analyst become angry. For example, the analyst might have been late or might have greeted the patient absent-mindedly. The patient now finds himself in the difficult position of wanting to talk about this, to restore a more harmonious relationship with the analyst, yet being afraid to do so, lest by mentioning it he alienate the analyst still more. In this dilemma, the patient may resort to a dream communication. He might then report a dream alluding to the distressing occurrence, omitting perhaps the person of the analyst from it. This makes it possible to make the dangerous communication while keeping the patient protected, since the analyst can interpret the dream in many different ways (Szasz, 1959c).

If the analyst is able and willing to accept the patient's reproach, he can so interpret the dream. Its covert communicative aim will then have been achieved: the important message was dispatched, the relationship to the analyst was not further endangered, and a more harmonious relationship between patient and analyst was established. On the other hand, if the analyst is upset, defensive, or otherwise unresponsive to the dream's hidden message, he might interpret the communication in some other way. Although this is clearly less desirable for the course of the analysis, it is preferable for the patient to making an overt accusation and being reprimanded for it. The misunderstanding at least does not place an additional burden on an already disharmonious relationship.

The idea that dreams are allusions is not new. Freud (1900, 1901) himself said this. However, he paid less attention to dream-communications as interpersonal events than he did to the intrapsychic aspects of dreaming. And in a short paper provocatively titled 'To Whom Does One Relate One's Dreams?' Ferenczi (1912) dealt explicitly with dreams as indirect communications.

Hysteria as Hinting

Any relatively non-discursive idiom may be used for hinting. Hence, communication by iconic body signs, as in hysteria, is well suited for hinting. Freud attributed the multiplicity of meanings characteristic of hysterical and other psychiatric symptoms to a 'motivational overdetermination'. In other words, he attributed the multiple meanings of dreams and symptoms – each meaning or interpretation having something to recommend it – to the multiplicity of (instinctual) motives which, he assumed, the final act (symptom) satisfied. In this study, the same phenomena are examined from a semiotical rather than from a motivational point of view. Accordingly, instead of an 'overdetermination of symptoms', I speak of a diversity of communicational meanings.

The hinting function of hysterical symptoms may be illustrated by the following example. Freud's patient Frau Cäcilie M. suffered from hysterical facial pain, which had at least two distinct meanings.

1. Its *overt meaning*, directed to the self, significant objects, physician, and others, was something like this: 'I am sick. You must help me! You must be good to me!' (The physician may have interpreted the message more specifically as: 'This is facial neuralgia, possibly tic douloureux.')

2. Its *covert meaning*, directed principally to a specific person (who may have been either an actual person, or an internal object, or both), may be paraphrased as follows: 'You have hurt me as if you had slapped my face. You should be sorry and make amends.'

Such communicational interactions are common between husbands and wives and between parents and children. This type of communication is fostered by social conditions rendering people closely interdependent for mutual need-satisfactions, requiring each person to curb his desires in order to satisfy any of them. Moreover, having curbed his needs, the person is in a better position to demand that his partner(s) do likewise. Thus, the open, undistorted expression of needs is discouraged, and various types of indirect communications and need-satisfactions are encouraged.

On the other hand, relatively open-ended social situations, for example those encountered in many phases of modern business life, foster relatively impersonal kinds of interdependence, based on *functional-instrumental factors. A supplies B's needs because of his special know-how, rather than because of a special relationship between them.*

Institutionally based, restrictive relationships, such as those among family members or professional colleagues, must be contrasted with instrumentally based, non-restrictive relationships serving the aims of practical (technologic, scientific, economic, etc.) pursuits, such as those between freely practising experts and their clients or between sellers and buyers. In instrumentally structured situations it is not necessary for the participants to curb their needs, because the mere expression of needs in no way compels others to gratify them, as it tends to do in the family (Szasz, 1959f). Indeed, not only is the frank expression of needs not inhibited, but it is often encouraged, since it helps to identify a 'problem' for which someone might have a 'solution'.

Two antithetical proverbs underscore these principles. One is the English saying that 'Honesty is the best policy.' The other is the Hungarian adage which, freely translated, warns: 'Tell the truth and you will get your head bashed in.' At first glance, these two proverbs express opposite messages. If treated simply as logical assertions, they are indeed contradictory. The conflict between them, however, is more apparent than real, because each maxim refers to a different social context. Honesty is, indeed, the best policy in instrumentally oriented human relationships and in the 'open' groups in which such activities flourish. Conversely, one will get his head bashed in for telling the truth, if one operates in an institutional setting or a 'closed' group. These principles may be illustrated by the fates of Galileo and Einstein. The former, operating in the institutional setting of the Roman Catholic Church, was punished for 'telling the truth'. The latter, operating in the instrumental setting of modern theoretical physics, was rewarded for it.

PART III
Rule-following Analysis of Behaviour

8 The Rule-following Model of Human Behaviour

Psychoanalysis has been correctly described as a motivational psychology: it offers explanations couched in terms of motives. According to Freud's earliest hypotheses concerning hysteria and other mental symptoms, a previously unrecognized motive was required to explain the patient's behaviour. For example, an obsessional symptom attributed by the patient to solicitude over his loved ones was interpreted as due to death wishes. Thus, one motive or goal, namely 'to do good' for someone, was replaced by another, namely 'to do harm'. It is clear, however, that although explanation in terms of motives is useful, it is insufficient for both psychological theory and psychoanalytic therapy. This is because motives tend to explain actions in a general or abstract sort of way. They do not really tell us why Mr Jones acted in a particular manner at a certain moment. To explain specific, concrete human actions, we must know other things besides what motivates the actor. The concepts of role and rule are indispensable in this connection.

Motives and Rules

In his essay, *The Concept of Motivation*, Peters (1958) explored the distinctions between psychological explanations couched in terms of motives as against those couched in terms of rule-following or purposive behaviour. Crucial to Peters's inquiry was his distinction between *action* and *happening*.

As I have emphasized earlier, this distinction is inherent in the psychoanalytic theory of 'mental illness' and is indispensable for differentiating – at least as regards therapeutic attitude – between physicochemical disorders of the body and so-called mental symptoms. The former are happenings or occurrences; developing carcinoma of the colon is an example. In contrast, so-called mental symptoms are doings or actions; for example, a hand-washing compulsion. Such 'mental symptoms' do not happen to one, but are (unconsciously) willed.

Peters also noted that to foresee and foretell what a person will do, it often is not necessary to know much about him as an individual. It is enough to know the role he is playing:

We know what the parson will do when he begins to walk towards the pulpit in the middle of the penultimate hymn or what the traveller will do when he enters the doors of the hotel because we know the *conventions* regulating church services and staying at hotels. *And we can make such predictions without knowing anything about the causes of people's behaviour. Man in society is like a chessplayer writ large.* ([Italics added] p. 7)

From this, Peters concluded that the first things that we must know about human actions are the norms and goals that regulate the actor's conduct. Accordingly, anthropology and sociology must be considered the basic sciences of human action, for these disciplines are concerned with exhibiting, in a systematic manner, the framework of norms and goals which are necessary to classify actions as being of a certain sort. Psychiatry and psychoanalysis, too, address themselves to these problems, although they often do so unwittingly. For example, in the psychoanalytic study of perversions or so-called antisocial acts, the observer is perforce concerned with norms and goals. By tacitly subscribing to the socially prevalent norms – as did Freud, for instance, in *Three Essays on the Theory of Sexuality* (1905b) – it may appear as if the author were *not* concerned with norms at all but only with 'psychosexual functions' (Szasz, 1959a).

On Causal and Conventional Explanations

What is the basis for distinguishing *causal from conventional explanations in psychology*? We encounter here, but in a new and more manageable form, the classical dichotomy between mechanistic causality and vitalistic teleology. In terms of our present inquiry, the distinction is between 'hidden-factor' explanations of behaviour as against 'convention' theories of it. The libido theory is a typical example of the former, while role theory exemplifies the latter. Hidden-factor theories, in common with the classic theories of physics, frame their explanatory statements in terms of antecedently acting events or forces (e.g. instincts, drives, libido, etc.). They try to explain the present and the future by what happened in the past. In contrast, rule-following explanations of behaviour are framed in terms of behaviour-regulating conventions. The relation of conventions to time must be explicitly specified. Obviously, many rules that governed conduct in the past no longer do now; others may have been active in the past, may still be active in the present, and may be expected to remain active in the foreseeable future; still others may be projected into the future. Hence, the future may influence conduct as much as – indeed even more than – the past.

What, then, is the difference between a causal and a rule-following type of explanation for a given bit of behaviour? According to Peters (1958), Freud was principally concerned with a general class of activities – composed of such things as dreams, obsessions, phobias, perversions, hallucinations, and so forth – characterized by the fact that they seemed 'to have no point or a very odd point' (p. 10). Freud reclaimed these phenomena for psychology 'by extending the model of purposive rule-following behaviour to cover the unconscious' (p. 11).

It is correct, therefore, to consider Freud's work, at least a part of it, a successful extension of the principle of rule-following to so-called unconsciously determined behaviour. This perspective is expressed most clearly in the psychoanalytic position towards personality change, for symptoms are treated *as if* they adhered to a rule-following pattern. Indeed, nowhere in psychoanalysis is there sufficient allowance made for a person who acts in a self-damaging way because he is stupid or ill-informed. Thus, rule-following explanations are not only accepted in psychoanalysis, but they are overemphasized and are applied in situations in which they do not and cannot fit.

The contrasting thesis – namely, that Freud proposed a mechanical-causal type of explanation for 'unconsciously determined' acts – is supported by the fact that he attributed 'neurotic' behaviour to such things as the repetition compulsion, the persistent operation of a repressed Oedipus complex, infantile fixations, the excessive strength of instincts or part-instincts, and so forth. Epistemologically, each of these constructs occupies a position similar to an antecedent physical occurrence. Many classical psychoanalytic explanations of behaviour have this cause-and-effect type of logical structure. The main reason for this probably was that Freud was ensnared in a moral dilemma from which he tried to extricate himself by means of ostensibly non-moral arguments. Like others in his social milieu, Freud equated 'conscious' rule-following behaviour with the notions of responsibility and punishability. Because he wished to treat hysteria (and mental illnesses generally) in a non-judge-mental and 'scientific' fashion, he had no choice but to deny and mystify the very discovery he had made – namely, that peculiar or symptomatic behaviour also obeys the principles of rule-following actions. His famous therapeutic dictum, 'Where id was, ego shall be', could be translated into our present idiom to mean that 'obscure and inexplicit rule-following shall be replaced by clear and deliberate rule-following'. In the following chapters the precise rules which hysterical behaviour follows, how such behaviour originates, and why it persists will be described and examined.

Nature and Convention – Biology and Sociology

A fundamental principle of modern science is that there is a *logical gulf* between nature and convention.[1] Adhering to this important distinction, Peters (1958) re-emphasized that 'move-ments *qua* movements are neither intelligent, efficient, nor correct. They only become so in the context of action' (p. 14). It follows, too, that whether a given phenomenon involving human participation is regarded as *action* or *happening* will have the most far-reaching consequences, because happenings 'cannot be characterized as intelligent or unintelligent, correct or in-correct, efficient or inefficient. Prima facie they are just occur-

[1] This distinction is completely obscured – or perhaps one should say suc-cessfully denied – in the religious conception of 'natural law'. According to Catholic doctrine, sexual behaviour *is (should be?)* regulated by 'natural law'.

rences' (p. 15). For occurrences or happenings, causal explanations are appropriate and conventional ones are not.

Finally, Peters noted that when a person is asked to state the motives for his actions, it is sometimes implied that he might be up to no good; and when it is said that his motives are unconscious, it is often implied further that he is not only up to no good but does not even *know* it! Accordingly, there is an important difference between giving a *reason* for one's action and giving a *justification* for it. Reasons and causes operate, so to speak, in an ethically neutral field, whereas motives and justifications are used in a context in which ethical considerations are explicitly or implicitly entertained.

A motive-analysis of mental illness thus functioned not merely as a scientific explanation but also, or perhaps primarily, as a justification both for the patient's behaviour and for the physician's interest in the patient and his efforts to help him.

Rules, Morals, and the Superego

The psychoanalytic concept of the superego must now be related to the notion of rule-following and to our ideas about ethics and morals. By ethics and morals we refer to the rules that men follow in the conduct of their lives, and sometimes also to the study of these rules (e.g. ethics as the study of moral conduct). The psychoanalytic concept superego refers to much the same things. We are confronted here with several words, some technical and others in common usage, all of which mean more or less the same thing. For the sake of clarity, it is best to speak simply of rule-following and of the consciousness of rules. In this way we can avoid several problems. For example, the word morality, as Peters (1958) noted, is not usually used to designate everyday, habitual acts or obsessive behaviour. It refers, rather, to the 'intelligent following of rules the point of which is understood' (p. 87). On the whole, Freud failed to deal explicitly with rule-following behaviour, except that based on the principle that men (children) obey feared and respected persons (adults). He had little to say concerning co-operative, mutually adjustive behaviour among equal adults.

This basic weakness of psychoanalytic theory stems from the fact that Freud was much more interested in pointing up the defects inherent in the 'morality of infantilism' than he was in defining what sort of morality is appropriate for an adult, fully socialized person.

Still, it would be erroneous to believe that psychoanalytic theory makes no contribution to describing and assessing different types of ethical conduct. The crucial notion in this connection is the relative rigidity or flexibility of the superego. The childish, immature, or 'neurotic' superego is rigid; it is characterized by slavish adherence to rules which, moreover, may not be clearly understood. The mature or 'normal' super-ego, on the other hand, is flexible; it can evaluate the situation at hand and modify the rules accordingly. According to an early, classic formulation (Strachey, 1934), the effectiveness of psycho-analysis as treatment depends upon the analyst's interventions (mutative interpretations) when these result in changing the patient's superego in the direction of greater flexibility. As far as it goes, this is a sound conception. However, like the psycho-analytic theory of the superego, it is severely limited by the fact that it is silent on what sort of rigidity is considered 'bad' and what sort of flexibility 'good'. In other words, *Freud and other psychoanalysts have persistently dallied with normative systems without ever committing themselves on normative standards.*

Indeed, when it came to confronting openly the issue of normative standards, Freud refused the challenge. He went so far as to reiterate the simple, common-sense belief that many people hold – namely, that 'right' is what they do:

Many years ago [Freud] conducted a private correspondence with Putnam on the subject of ethics. Putnam showed it to me and I remember these two sentences: Ich betrachte das Moralische als etwas Selbstversändliches . . . Ich habe eigentlich nie etwas Gemeines getan. (Jones, 1957; p. 247)

Now, to say that morality is self-evident and to believe that one had never done a mean thing are peculiar statements to come from the lips of a scientist whose object of study was man, himself included. It reflects, I believe, Freud's determination to exclude this area from critical examination.

Since psychoanalysis deals predominantly with learned behaviour, considerations of norms or standards are always pertinent to the adequate formulation and explanation of its observations. Indeed, it would be difficult to overemphasize the fact that virtually all behaviour with which the psychologist deals is learned. The concept of learning is, moreover, operationally tied to the concept of performance. One learns how to act in order to measure up to norms or achieve goals. Both learning and performance presuppose standards of correctness; the notion of performance is thus fundamental to the sociologist's view of human behaviour (Goffman, 1959).

Rules, Roles, and Personal Commitment

Sometimes the line of demarcation between happening and action is not clear. The point at which a passively incurred event becomes transformed into a role-playing situation, provided that the person involved is neurologically intact, will depend on his own attitude towards his human condition. By 'attitude' I refer to such things as whether he is hopeful or dejected, oriented towards patterns of active mastery or passive endurance, and so forth. Consider, for example, the hypothetical case of a man who is involved in a train collision on his way to work. Injured and rendered temporarily unconscious, he is taken to a hospital. All this happens to him. On regaining consciousness he finds himself in the patient role. From this moment on, his behaviour – or at least some aspects of it – can and must be analysed in terms of rule-following and role-playing. Indeed, no other analysis could adequately account for his personal conduct once his total passivity due to unconsciousness is replaced by a measure of awareness. While this may be obvious, I emphasize it because people in quandaries often regard themselves as utterly helpless, the 'victims of circumstances'.

Of course, people may or may not be victims of circumstances. Usually, unfavourable circumstances and personal 'styles of life' (A. Adler, 1931) both play a role in shaping the fates of men. The point is that even though a person may experience and define his situation as if he played no part in bringing it about, this may in fact not be true. On the contrary, such a claim often serves a defensive purpose. In other words, when choices are made – either by specific action, or more often by inaction – and when these lead to unhappy consequences, people often feel that 'it was not their fault' that things turned out as they did. In a purely conventional moral sense they might be correct. But this is simply because common sense assigns guilt or blame only to the specific commission of acts – much less often to omissions – and even among these usually only to acts whose deleterious effects are immediate or short range. In any case, I would insist that, to some extent at least, all people shape their own destiny, no matter how much they might bewail the superior forces of alien wills and powers.

Rules and Anti-rules

To assert that man is a rule-following animal implies more than that he is inclined to act on the basis of rules which he has been taught. He is also inclined to act in diametrical opposition to these rules.

In this connection, Freud's (1910b) observations concerning the antithetical meanings of so-called primal words are pertinent. He noted that certain basic words of a language may be used to express contrary meanings; in Latin, for example, *sacer* means holy and accursed. This antithetical meaning of symbolism is an important characteristic of dream psychology. In a dream, a symbol may stand for itself or for its opposite – for example, tall may signify tall or short, or young may stand for young or old. I have suggested (Szasz, 1957a, pp. 162–3) that this principle also applies to affects. Illustrative examples are feeling afraid, which may signify that one is vigilant and prepared for danger; or feeling guilty, which may signify that one is conscientious. This antithetical signification seems to be inherent in the nature of man's capacity to form and use symbols of all types. It applies to affects, iconic signs, words, rules, and systems of rules (games), each of which may signify or, more often, suggest both the referent and its opposite.

Anti-rules are especially significant in the behaviour of psychosocially simple (immature) persons. Thus children and simple, poorly educated persons tend to structure and perceive their world mainly in terms of the rules they have been given plus their opposites. Although it is possible to modify rules or to construct new ones, to do so requires some sophistication. Hence, this option is not available to young children or, unfortunately, to many adults. It must be emphasized, too, that while positive rule-following tends to assure interpersonal and social harmony, it alone often fails to satisfy the human needs for personal autonomy and integrity. To satisfy these needs it is necessary to follow one's own rules. *The simplest rules which we experience as our own are anti-rules.* Thus, as early as during the first year of life, when babies are urged to eat, they learn to protest by refusing to eat. The so-called negativism of young children probably constitutes the earliest instances of following anti-rules. This is well understood by intuitive persons and is expressed by such remarks as 'If I want him to do something, I must ask him to do the opposite.' The proverbially stubborn mule can be made to advance only if his master acts as if he were trying to make him back up. We touch here on the immense subject of doing something because it is forbidden, the significance of which in delinquent or antisocial behaviour has already received much attention from psychiatrists and psychologists. The notion of anti-rules delineated here, however, is of somewhat wider scope since it pertains equally to prescriptive and prohibitive rules.

Consider, for instance, the rules given in the Ten Commandments. Some are prohibitions – for example, of murder and theft. Others are prescriptions – for example, to honour one's father and mother. Clearly, each of these implies and suggests its opposite. To be told not to kill creates the idea that one might kill. It might be objected that people had this and similar ideas before the Ten Commandments were promulgated, and that most laws are aimed at curbing propensities that exist prior to legislation. This is true. Still, it does not negate the fact that laws – especially some modern laws – also create and encourage propensities towards certain forms of behaviour. Given the common human inclination to disobey laws – 'Forbidden fruit tastes sweeter', as the proverb has it – any law might create an incentive for men to act in opposition to it.

A Classification of Rules

We are ready to examine the function and transmission of rules. Children growing up in contemporary Western cultures must learn a large variety of rules. These may be conveniently divided into three classes: (1) natural laws or biological rules; (2) prescriptive laws or social (religious, moral) rules; and (3) imitative or interpersonal rules.

Biological Rules

Biological rules form a special part of the larger category commonly called the Laws of Nature. These rules are concerned with the physics and chemistry of the human body in relation to its material or non-human environment. The implicit aim of biological rules – made explicit by man – is survival of the individual as a body or physical machine and survival of the species as a biological system. Many basic biological rules are learned by direct experience, but some, at least in a rudimentary form, may be said to be inborn. More sophisticated knowledge concerning biological rules must be learned by the methods of science. Indeed, the basic medical sciences could be said to be devoted to this end.

In this connection, the question arises as to whether animals 'know' certain basic biological rules. In one sense, the answer must be that they do, for without 'obeying' them they would perish. It is important, however, to be clear about the sense in which animals 'know' such rules. This knowledge consists of the appropriate responses to certain objects in their environment; it is automatic, conditioned, and not self-reflective. In a hierarchy of learning and knowing, this type of knowledge would have to be considered the simplest and most basic. It consists of responding to objects as objects, not as signs, and may be called object-learning.

Usually, animals do not know any other types of rules (meta-rules). Although some monkeys play games, and many animals can readily be taught to follow rules by imitation and practice (dancing bears, ball-balancing seals, etc.), it appears that the animal's limited capacity for symbolization restricts his use of rules to those which are non-reflective. In other words, animals cannot use rules intelligently, possessing an awareness or knowledge that they are using rules. This may be inferred from the fact that animals cannot readily modify rules in accordance with the exigencies of a particular situation, nor can they usually create new patterns of rules (new games). Thus animals cannot learn metarules and cannot play metagames.[2]

Social, Religious, or Moral Rules

In the class of social, religious, and moral rules belong all prescriptive laws governing social relationships, whether these are said to originate from a single God, a multiplicity of deities, or culture and society. These laws differ from so-called natural laws with respect to geographical scope or distribution and also in the nature of the sanctions. Natural laws hold for all parts of the world, although, as it is now realized, they may not apply in situations outside of it, for example on another planet.

The term 'social rules' designates all the rules that originate from the prevailing practices of a social group. If these are significantly disobeyed, the *person* will perish. Emphasis here is on the word 'person', for our focus has shifted from biological to social survival. Social survival depends on adapting to the social rules or changing them to suit one's needs, much as biological survival depends on adapting to biological rules.

Imitative or Interpersonal Rules

Imitative or interpersonal rules are learned, principally in childhood, by imitating someone else's example. Illustrative are the innumerable instances in which *children look*, literally as well as metaphorically, to their parents, siblings, or peers, *to see how they should act*. Their conduct is thus based on example, much as a mock-up model in engineering serves as an example after which the products to be manufactured are fashioned.

The boundary between imitative and social rules may not always be sharp or clear. Some social rules are acquired by

[2] A systematic discussion of rule- and game-hierarchies will be presented in Chapter 11.

imitation. Moreover, since imitative rules are learned chiefly in the family, they really form a subgroup of the larger class called 'social rules'. Nevertheless, it is useful – especially for our present purpose in regard to hysteria and mental illness – to draw as sharp a distinction as possible between these two types of rules. Let us therefore pay special attention to the differences between social and interpersonal rules.

Imitative rules usually refer to trivial, everyday matters, such as how to eat, dress, care for one's body, and so forth. These rules are usually not spelled out in verbal form. Instead of being explicitly stated, they are exhibited in the actual everyday behaviour of the older members of the family or group. Children acquire these rules by 'blind imitation'. The 'blind' quality of this learning process must be emphasized, because in contrast to, say, attempting to forge another person's signature – this type of imitation is unconscious or unreflective. In learning one's mother tongue, for instance, one is not aware of imitating other people.

In contrast to the trivial nature of many of the acts learned by imitative rule-following, and to the inexplicit nature of these rules, social rules refer to the regulation of more important behavioural situations governed by explicitly stated rules. In other words, while imitative rules refer to customs, social rules articulate moral-religious prescriptions or secular laws. The sanctions for each vary correspondingly. Failure to learn or comply with imitative rules leads merely to being thought of as eccentric, stupid, foolish, or naughty. Deviance from social rules, however, brings serious consequences upon the offender, ranging from being labelled bad or guilty to expulsion from family (or group), or even to loss of life. By and large, sociologists have concentrated their attention on social rules; psychologists and especially psychoanalysts have focused on imitative or interpersonal rules; and anthropologists have been most attentive to all of these. (See Table 5 for a schematic summary of the characteristics of these three types of rules.)

TABLE 5. THREE TYPES OF RULES: BIOLOGICAL, SOCIAL, AND INTERPERSONAL

	Biological Rules	Social Rules	Interpersonal Rules
Example	'You must eat to live; otherwise you will starve to death.'	'You must worship God to live; otherwise you will be expelled from the group.'	'If you are a male, you must grow up to be self-reliant, so that you can provide for your wife and children; otherwise you will not be able to consider yourself a grown man.'
Subject-matter studied by Aims of the rules	Biological sciences Survival of physical body and/or species. Biological identity	Sociology, anthropology Survival of (large) group as a social organization. Social (group) identity	Psychology, psychoanalysis Survival of small group (family) or individual, as social being. Individual identity
Sanctions for breaking the rules	1. Illness or disability of the body 2. Dissolution of the physical body: 'biological death'	Socially deviant behaviour and 'punishment': 'crime', 'sin' 1. Expulsion from the group; loss of social identity; social death	Interpersonally conflictful behaviour; personal defeat, frustration, and unhappiness; 'mental illness', 'human failure'
Sanctions codified as	Natural laws	Legal (or religious) 'laws'	Customs, standards of personal behaviour
Rewards for successfully modifying the rules	Extension of life span and increase in physical effectiveness and health	Enlarged scope of human fraternity and co-operation (e.g. supranational versus national interests and identity)	Creative self-determination; enhanced sense of identity and freedom
Rate of change	Nil or very slow	Gradual	Most rapid

The Need for Rules

The existence and durability of social rules – irrespective of the sources to which man may have attributed them – is evidence of the intensity of the human need to follow rules. Indeed, man's need for rules and his propensity to follow them is equalled only by his burning ambition to be free of rules. As I will try to show later, this antithetical attitude is a special instance of a more general human proclivity – namely, the need for intimacy and the simultaneous need for solitude. Oscillating attitudes of submission to and rebellion against people and rules may be best viewed as manifestations of this fundamental human paradox. In our efforts to resolve this dilemma, one of the most useful methods at our disposal is the human capacity for abstraction which makes it possible to construct progressively higher levels of symbolization; these constructs, in turn, lead to a lessening of the feeling of compulsion attached to all rules explicitly understood *as* rules. Thus, for each set of rules we can, in principle, construct a set of metarules. The latter are made up of the specifications governing the formation of the rules at the next lower (logical) level. Explicit awareness of metarules implies an understanding of the origin, function, and scope of the (next lower-level) rules. The acquisition of such understanding is a form of *mastery*. Only by practising what may be called the metarule attitude – which is actually a special case of the scientific attitude applied to the domain of rules – can a secure yet flexible integration of rules as behaviour-regulating agencies be achieved. Finally, the metarule attitude makes it possible to increase the range of choices concerning whether or not and how to comply with rules, whether or not and how to change them, and the limits and consequences of our decisions about these matters.

9 The Ethics of Helplessness and Helpfulness

I suggested that 'hysteria' refers to the expression and communication – chiefly by means of non-verbal, bodily signs – of a state of disability or 'illness'. The implicit aim of the communication is to secure help. If the problem of hysteria is framed in this way, it becomes logical to ask: Where did the idea originate that the rules of the game of life ought to be so defined that those who are weak, disabled, or ill should be helped? The first answer is that this is the game usually played in childhood: every one of us was a weak and helpless child, and was cared for by adults; without such help we would not have survived to adulthood.

The second general answer to this question is that the rules prescribing a help-giving attitude towards the weak – that is, the rules characteristic of the child–parent interaction or of the family game – derive from the dominant religions of Western man. Judaism, and especially Christianity, teach these rules. They do so by means of myth, example, exhortation, and whenever possible by the use of appropriate negative sanctions.

This chapter will be devoted to an exposition of the nature and actual psychosocial operation of these two general systems of rules. The first could be regarded as the rules of the family game; the second, those of the religious game. I singled out these rules for consideration because they provide, in part, the psychosocial basis and the continuing rationale for so-called hysterical behaviour as well as for certain other 'mental illnesses'. In short, *men learn how to be 'mentally ill' by following (mainly) the rules of these two games.*[1] Since ethical systems

[1] The basic premise which underlies my attempt to formulate a coherent theory of personal conduct is that it is always, at least in part, an expression of *learning and human creativity*. This approach to psychiatry is anything but

consist basically of rules of social conduct that men are enjoined to follow, the two systems which will be considered may properly be regarded as constituting the ethics of helplessness and helpfulness.

Childhood and the Rules of Helplessness

Freud emphasized repeatedly that man's prolonged childhood was responsible for his proneness to develop what he called 'neurosis'. The idea that childishness is somehow related to 'mental illness' (as well as to misbehaviours of all sorts) is obviously very old. The main shortcomings of this notion are its generality and vagueness. To be useful, whether for psychological theory or for psychotherapy, the precise details of the common human tendency to remain childish, or to reassume childish patterns of behaviour must be elucidated.

Regression versus Infantilization

Freud's basic thesis was that man *wanted* to remain a child and was driven forward, as it were, only by forces generated by instinctual (sexual) frustration. And this frustration he saw as coming from 'culture'. He thus postulated an irreconcilable conflict between the interests of instinctual and especially sexual satisfaction on the one hand, and cultural, including social, needs and development on the other (Freud, 1927, 1930). Implicit in this position is the postulate that man's tendency to remain immature is 'biologically given'. Regression is thus considered to satisfy a 'need' similar to the biologically determined needs for water, food, or sexual activity. This view, which provides a quasi-biological explanation for the tendency to regress, makes it unnecessary to search for social factors which might contribute to this type of behaviour. In recent decades, numerous students of man have taken issue with this theory of

novel. It received its initial impetus from Freud and Pavlov and was subsequently carried forward by A. Adler (1907–37), Dollard and Miller (1941, 1950), Fromm (1941, 1947), Goldstein (1951), Horney (1939), Jung (1940), Sullivan (1947, 1953), and others.

'human nature'. One of the most searching objections to it we owe to Susanne Langer (1942).

In my view there are no good grounds for accepting the view that man desires the *status quo* and is driven forward only by privation, culture, or what not. In fact, this formulation seems to be merely a new, more scientific-sounding, version of the ancient biblical story of man's fall from divine grace – of Adam and Eve's expulsion from the Garden of Eden. The very fact that God forbade these two 'original sinners' ever to return to the Garden implied that they wanted to return. For if Adam and Eve did not wish to return to Paradise, how would they have been punished? The traditional psychoanalytic theory of human growth likewise postulates that *regressive goals are primary*. Sublimation is considered a poor substitute; one, it is implied, that would be relinquished instantly if the original regressive goals were rendered (unconflictfully) attainable.

I submit that 'Paradise Lost' is still another myth. The pleasurable qualities of childhood experiences and of regressive goals generally have been vastly overrated. Dispensing with the whole vexing problem of precisely how happy or satisfying childhood gratifications are, I shall adhere, instead, to a position concerning human psychosocial maturation essentially similar to Langer's. However, I wish to supplement her basic thesis, that man has a need for symbolization and symbolic expression, by adding two complementary notions to it: firstly, that man has a primary (further irreducible) need for object contact or human relationships; secondly, that the notions of objects, symbols, rules, and roles are intimately connected, so that man's growth towards personal identity and integrity on the one hand, and towards social tolerance and decreasing need for group narcissism on the other, go hand in hand with increasing sophistication in regard to the understanding and use of symbols, rules, roles, and games (Szasz, 1957c). I believe, therefore, that the seemingly basic human tendency to remain childish and to strive for so-called regressive goals is not necessarily biologically given but may be better explained along the following lines.

Learning *is* difficult. It requires effort, diligence, self-discipline, perseverance, and so forth. Persistence in habitual patterns of behaviour is, at the very least, labour-saving.

However valid this principle might be – and I do not wish to minimize its significance – its relevance depends on a scarcity of zest and interest in the learner. Should a person be healthy and energetic – that is to say, should he be psychologically affluent – then the principle that saving effort is a 'good thing' will no longer apply. Such a person, much as an energetic and economically productive society, will need to produce and consume rather than only to conserve. The need to save psychological 'labour' is, therefore, not a general law of psychology. Indeed, this 'need' emerges only under certain unfavourable conditions such as fatigue, ill health, stupidity, or social circumstances which discourage or prohibit learning.

I believe that the significance of religious, social, and personal prohibitions placed on knowledge and learning have been surprisingly underestimated in most scientific theories of man. By way of illustration, let us consider the following examples:

1. Jewish and Christian religions attribute man's fall from divine grace to Adam's having partaken of the fruit of the tree of knowledge.

2. The Roman Catholic Church used to list books (and other materials, such as films) which were prohibited for members of this faith.

3. Many other more subtle, but equally powerful, social forces prevent people from learning certain facts about biology, or pharmacology, or other people's religious beliefs or national customs. All sorts of national narcissisms and racial prejudice, no less than religious beliefs and teachings, encourage and reward various forms of covert infantilism.

4. Finally, certain individuals, acting in specific relationships to others, foster non-learning behaviour in their partners – for example, the parent who rewards his child's persistent helplessness and dependency in order to enhance his own importance and self-esteem. This sort of occurrence is extremely common.

The Rule : 'The Sick and the Sufferer Must Be Helped!'

Like the infant's cry, the message 'I am sick' is exceedingly effective in mobilizing others to some kind of helpful action. In accordance with this communicative impact of sickness, physicians – following in the footsteps of their predecessors, the priests – often define their occupation as a 'calling'. This implies that it is not only the sick and helpless who are *calling* them, but God as well. The helpers thus hasten to the side of the helpless – the sick or disabled – and minister to him to restore him to health. In this imagery, the role of the helpless or sick person is so defined that he is entitled to help simply *because* he is disabled. If we do not help him, especially if we could, we incur moral blame for our neglect.

It often happens that this game of helpfulness is played so that those who want to give help unwittingly obligate themselves to caring for those who want to get help. They no longer choose to offer or withhold help, depending on circumstances, but instead are committed to an unwritten contract that soon becomes quite burdensome for them. It is no wonder, then, that if a person is found to malinger, his behaviour may be experienced by those on the help-giving team as if it were a form of blackmail. Physicians react to such persons in much the same way as we all would if confronted by an individual holding a contract extremely injurious to us which he was trying to enforce with all the power at his command. Although Freud never dealt with this problem in these terms, he was well aware of it and was prepared to face it in the tradition of rationalism. This may be inferred from his insistence that the financial aspects of the patient–physician relationship be openly discussed (Freud, 1913, p. 346). Until then – and often even today – physicians were not in the habit of speaking of money matters with patients. This behaviour served several purposes, among them the wish to avoid interfering with the image of the sick–helper relationship sketched above. To preserve the belief that the sick receive medical help because they *need it*, it is necessary to deny the fact that they pay for it. The possibility that attitudes of 'kindness' towards 'poor patients' serve, by and large, the purpose of enhancing the doctor's self-esteem must be concealed at all cost.

We must scrutinize, therefore, all therapeutic attitudes traditionally ascribed to benevolence, keeping always in mind that such manoeuvres on the part of the therapist may serve only to depreciate and subjugate the patient. We may recall, in this connection, the relationship between the slave-owner and his Negro slave. The master treated his servant 'kindly' – often perhaps more kindly than was the Negro in a northern industrial jungle, as white supremacists are still eager to point out. But this very benevolence and paternalism were a part of the code of slavery.

Similarly, much of what passes for 'medical ethics' is a set of paternalistic rules the net effect of which is the persistent infantilization and domination of the patient by the physician. A shift towards greater dignity, freedom, and self-responsibility for the disenfranchised – whether slave, sinner, or patient – can be secured only at the cost of honest and serious commitment to an ethic of autonomy and egality. This implies that all persons are treated with respect, consideration, and dignity. While accorded the opportunities for more decent human relationships, the formerly disenfranchised must, at the same time, be expected to shoulder certain responsibilities, among them the responsibility to be maximally self-reliant and responsible even when ill or disabled.

Herbert Spencer on Helping the Helpless

Herbert Spencer, often considered one of the founders of modern sociology, was profoundly interested in the problem of helping the helpless. Under the influence of Darwin's evolutionary conceptions of biology, he tried to base sociological principles on biological observations. Although this method is full of pitfalls, Spencer's views still deserve serious consideration.

Spencer presented his basic thesis that 'conformity . . . to two radically opposed principles [on which] the continuance of every higher species of creature depends' (p. 78) most completely in his essay *The Man Versus The State* (1884). In the case of every higher species of animal, wrote Spencer, 'the early lives of its members and the adult lives of its members have to be dealt with in contrary ways' (p. 78). He noted that animals of 'superior types' are comparatively slow in reaching maturity; having matured, however, they are able 'to give more aid to their offspring than animals of inferior types' (p. 78). He thereupon formulated the general law that 'during immaturity, benefits received must be inversely as the power or ability of the receiver. Clearly, if during his first part of life benefits were proportioned to merits, or rewards to deserts, the species would disappear in a generation' (p. 79).

Spencer then proceeded to contrast the 'regime of the family group' with the 'regime of that larger group formed by the adult members of the species' (p. 79). At some point in their lives, mature animals are left to themselves – to fulfil the requirements of life or to perish:

Now there comes into play a principle just the reverse of that above described. *Throughout the rest of its life, each adult gets benefit in proportion to merit, reward in proportion to desert:* merit and desert in each case being understood as ability to fulfil all the requirements of life – to get food, to secure shelter, or to escape enemies. Placed in competition with members of its own species and in antagonism with members of other species, it dwindles and gets killed off or thrives and propagates, according as it is ill-endowed or well-endowed ... The broad fact then, here to be noted, is that *Nature's modes of treatment inside the family-group and outside the family-group are diametrically opposed to one another*; and that the intrusion of either mode into the sphere of the other, would be fatal to the species either immediately or remotely. ([Italics added] pp. 79–80)

Spencer insisted that men can no more flout this Law of Nature than can animals. While he thought it necessary, and therefore proper, that children should be sheltered by their families, he felt strongly that a similar arrangement with respect to adults would bring disaster on the human species. In the true spirit of rugged individualism, Spencer pleaded for the self-reliant responsibility of man as opposed to the ministrations of the paternalistic state.

Surely none can fail to see that were the principle of family life to be adopted and fully carried out in social life – were reward always great in proportion as desert was small, fatal results to the society would quickly follow; and if so, then even a partial intrusion of the family regime into the regime of the state, will be slowly followed by fatal results. *Society, in its corporate capacity, cannot without immediate or remoter disaster interfere with the play of these opposed principles under which every species has reached such fitness for its mode of life as it possesses, and under which it maintains that fitness.* ([Italics added] p. 80)

I do not believe that quite such a direct application of biological principles to the social – and hence inherently ethical –

affairs of man is ever justified. I cite Spencer's views not so much for their political implications, as for their historical significance. Spencer was a senior contemporary of Freud's. His thesis concerning the significance, especially for social organization, of the basic biological relationship between parent and young became a cornerstone of psychoanalytic theory. Roheim (1943) created an elaborate anthropological theory of man based on essentially nothing more than a Spencerian notion of prolonged foetalization.

Although Spencer's argument is plausible, we must be careful lest we use it to explain too much. Emphasizing the human infant's biologically determined dependence on its parents in order to explain 'neurosis' may be a reversal of cause and effect. It seems probable that the human child remains dependent for so long not because his prolonged childhood is biologically determined, but because it takes him *a long time to learn all the symbols, rules, roles, and games which he must master before he can be considered a fully grown human being* (and not merely a biologically mature organism)!

Let us now reconsider the similarities, from a sociopsychological point of view, between being young (or immature) and being disabled (by illness or otherwise). For practical tasks, such as gathering food, building shelter, fighting off enemies, and so forth, children are useless. In fact, they are liabilities. The physically disabled, or those who, for whatever reason, refuse to play the game – by refusing to work – are similarly useless to society, and in fact constitute a liability for it. Why, then, do human societies tolerate persons with such disabilities? Evidently, because societies have concerns other than those for which disabled individuals are useless.

Because disabled adults are functionally similar to children, they fall readily into the same type of relationship to the able as children do to their parents. The disabled need help and will not survive without it. The able are capable of providing help and are motivated to do so. Besides the biologically built-in tendencies which parents may have to provide for their children (and for others in need), there are often socially given incentives promoting succouring behaviour. In primitive social groups, for example, children could be counted on to assist, just as soon as they were able, with the physical toils necessary for survival. Thus, caring for them when they were weak meant gaining helpers and allies when they were stronger.

The weakest link in Spencer's argument is his failure to make allowance for the fundamental change in man from *biological organism* to *social being*. With respect to the rule of helping those in need, this transformation means a change from acting automatically – that is, in conformity with biologically built-in mechanisms, triggered perhaps by environmental conditions – to becoming self-reflective, that is, aware of the rules themselves. Rules may be 'followed' regardless of which of these attitudes is maintained towards them. In the first instance, they are followed in an obligatory manner, for the person or animal has no opportunity to deviate from them. In contrast, self-reflective rule-following provides an opportunity to make choices – that is, to obey or disobey the rules. Moreover, awareness of the rules leads to a fresh condition – namely, the deliberate imitation of occurrences designed to bring the operation of the desired rules into play. Thus, as soon as men became intelligent, sign-using animals and hence aware of the kinds of relationships that invariably obtain between children and parents, the stage was set to imitate childishness to gain certain ends. The stage for the genesis of hysteria, too, was set at this early phase of human social development. The necessary conditions for the development of hysteria are, firstly, the biologically determined but socially implemented rule that parents (or well-functioning individuals) care for their children (or for ill-functioning individuals); and secondly, man's growth to self-reflection and awareness, made possible by the development of speech and symbolization. From this perspective, hysteria appears to be a creative – in a sense, progressive – development, rather than merely a disability or 'regression'.

Biblical Rules Fostering Disability and Illness

Jewish and Christian religious teachings abound in rules that reward sickness, malingering, poverty, fearfulness – in brief, disabilities of all sorts. Moreover, these rules, or their corollaries, invoke penalties for self-reliance, competence, effectiveness, and pride in health and well-being. This is a bold assertion, although not a particularly novel one. I shall try to support it by citing adequate evidence. I wish to emphasize that it is *not* my thesis that prescriptions fostering disability constitute the whole or the essence of the Bible. Taken in its entirety, the Bible is a complex and heterogeneous work, from which many diverse rules of conduct may be inferred. Indeed, the history of Western religions and morals illustrates how, by taking one or another part of this work, it is possible to support a wide variety of social or moral courses of action.

Personally, I espouse respect for the autonomy and integrity of one's self and others. No attempt to justify or support these values will be made here. I believe, however, that in a work of this kind it is necessary to make one's point of view towards such matters clear, to enable the reader to make allowances for or to correct the author's bias.

My approach to religious rules and behaviour is socio-psychological, not theological. Thus, whether my interpretations of religious rules are 'theologically accurate' is largely irrelevant. What is relevant is whether I have inferred correctly or falsely from the actual behaviour of persons professing to be religious the rules that govern and explain their conduct.

In addressing myself to scriptural passages as written statements, my position is that of a logically critical interpreter. I shall be critical of certain biblical rules, but in doing so shall be concerned less with condemning them than with making explicit the values they codify as worth striving for. Naturally, my interpretations will conflict with the interpretations of the modern clergyman trying to make scriptural texts fit for present-day consumption. It seems to me that so-called liberal interpretations of religious documents (whether Christian or Jewish) serve the aim of selling religion to modern man. It should not surprise us if vendors wrap up their merchandise so as to make it most attractive for the buyer – in this case, so that it will conflict as little as possible with the scientific and democratic aspects of modern Western civilization.

The motif that God loves the humble, the meek, the needy, or those who fear him is a thread running through both the Old and New Testaments. The idea that man should not be too well off lest he offend God is deeply ingrained in the Jewish religion. It was also present in classical Greek pantheism. Indeed, this element seems to be a part of most primitive religions, according to which man conceives of God in his own image: God is like man, only more so. God, then, is a kind of superman with his own needs for self-esteem and status and it is these privileges that mortal men are enjoined to respect. The Greek legend of Polycrates, the overly lucky king of Samos, illustrates this theme (Schiller, 1798).

This attitude, which is basically a dread of happiness generated by a powerful fear of envy, is fundamental to the psychology of the person seriously committed to the Judaeo-Christian ethic. The defensive, self-protective character of this 'masochistic' manoeuvre is evident. For such a tactic to be effective, it is necessary to assume, firstly, the presence of another person (or persons) and, secondly, the operation of certain rules by which this person conducts himself.

Who is man's partner-opponent in this game of 'I-am-not-happy'? What are the specific rules of this game that make this defence possible? As to the identity of the opponent, we may say, without going into unnecessary details, that it is God and a succession of other powerful figures vis-à-vis whom the player occupies a subservient position. The power differential between the two players is crucial, for it alone can account for the fear of envy. In a strong–weak relationship, only the weak member of the pair needs to fear arousing the envy of his partner. The strong has no such fears, because he knows that the weak is powerless to act destructively towards him.

In general, then, the open acknowledgement of satisfaction is feared only in situations of relative oppression – for example, all-suffering wife vis-à-vis domineering husband. *The experience and expression of satisfaction (joy, contentment) are inhibited lest they lead to an augmentation of one's burden.* This dilemma must be faced, for example, by persons who come from large, poor families and do moderately well financially while the other family members remain poor. If such a person manages to become very wealthy, he will be able to take care of all the other family members who want to be dependent on him. However, should he be only moderately well off, he will be faced with the threat that, irrespective of how hard he works, the demands of his poor relatives will prevent him from getting ahead. Their needs will always be greater than his assets. (Progressive taxation may create similar feelings in people.) If our hypothetical moderately successful man wants to prevent antagonizing his needy relatives, he will be prompted to 'malinger' in regard to his financial situation. By misrepresenting his economic affairs, he will try to protect himself from being 'robbed' of the fruits of his labours.

There is thus a close similarity between misrepresenting health as illness on the one hand, and wealth as poverty on the other. Although, on the surface, both manoeuvres seem painful and self-damaging, careful inspection of the total human situation in which they occur reveals that they are defensive operations. Their purpose is to sacrifice a part to save the whole. For example, in wartime, bodily survival may be safeguarded by simulating ill-health. Financial possessions may, in times of burdensome taxation, be similarly safeguarded by pretending to be poor.

The fear of acknowledging satisfaction is a characteristic feature of slave psychology. The 'properly exploited' slave is forced to labour until he shows signs of fatigue or exhaustion. Completion of his task does not signify that his work is finished and that he may rest. On the contrary, it only invites further demands. At the same time, even though his task is unfinished, he may be able to influence his master to stop driving him – and to let him rest – if he exhibits signs of imminent collapse. Such signs may be genuine or contrived. Exhibiting signs of fatigue or exhaustion – irrespective of whether they are genuine or contrived – is likely to induce a feeling of fatigue or exhaustion in the actor. I believe that this explains many of the so-called chronic fatigue states of which harassed people complain. Many such persons are unconsciously 'on strike' against individuals (actual or internal) to whom they relate subserviently and against whom they wage an unceasing and unsuccessful covert rebellion. In contrast to the slave, a free man sets, as far as he can, his own tempo of work. He can stop before becoming fatigued; and he can enjoy the fruits of his labours.

Let us now consider the particular rules that make disability or illness potential assets. In certain situations, the rules of the game prescribe that when man (subject, son, patient) is healthy, self-reliant, rich, and proud, then God (king, father, physician) shall be strict, demanding, even punitive. But should man be sick, help-seeking, poor, and humble, then God will care for him and protect him: God will forgive him, help him, love him, and allow him to be passive and incompetent. It might seem that I have exaggerated this rule. I do not believe so. Rather, this impression reflects our spontaneous antagonism to such a rule when it is clearly and forcefully stated.

Many biblical passages could be cited to support this thesis. In Luke (18:22–5) we read:

Now when Jesus heard these things, he said unto him, Yet lackest thou one thing: sell all that thou hast, and distribute unto the poor, and thou shalt have treasure in heaven: and come, follow me. And when he heard this, he was very sorrowful: for he was very rich. And when Jesus saw that he was very sorrowful, He said, How hardly shall they that have riches enter into the kingdom of God! For it is easier for a camel to go through a needle's eye, than for a rich man to enter into the kingdom of God.

The Sermon on the Mount (Matthew 5:1–12) is probably the best-known illustration of the rules fostering dependency and disability. Here, Jesus blesses the poor in spirit, the meek, the mourner, and so forth. This passage most clearly enunciates the basic rules by which the Christian God may be said to play his game with man. What does God pledge himself to do? And what type of behaviour is demanded of man? To formulate my answers, I have transformed and paraphrased the Beatitudes. Firstly, the biblical phrasing 'blessed are' has been translated into 'should'. Secondly, each positive injunction so obtained was supplemented by its corollary, framed in the form of a prohibition. The Beatitudes then read (in part) as follows:

The biblical text	*Its logical corollary*
(Matthew 5:3, 5, 8)	(My interpretation)
Blessed *are* the poor in spirit: for theirs is the kingdom of heaven.	Man should be 'poor in spirit' – i.e., stupid, submissive: Do not be smart, well-informed, or assertive!
Blessed *are* the meek: for they shall inherit the earth.	Man should be 'meek' – i.e., passive, weak, submissive: Do not be self-reliant!
Blessed *are* the pure in heart: for they shall see God.	Man should be 'pure in heart' – i.e., naïve, unquestioningly loyal: Do not entertain doubt (about God)!

Stated in this form, it is evident that these rules constitute a simple reversal of rules governing human rewards and punishments in life on earth. In this process of rule reversal, deficiencies in endowment, skill, and knowledge – or, in general, incompetence – have become codified as positive values. Elsewhere (Matthew 6:34), man is explicitly enjoined to 'take no thought for the morrow'. In other words, man should not plan for the future. He should not try to provide for himself and for those who depend on him. Instead, he should cultivate trust and faith in God. This is a reasonable rule for children, since in fact they cannot – and, if they have a father or a mother, need not – provide for themselves.

But what are the implications of these rules when espoused for and by adult men and women? These are the rules of irresponsibility and childish dependency. It is difficult to exaggerate the conflict between these rules and the demands of living according to the rules of autonomy, rationality, and self-responsibility. It remains a matter of conjecture, however, to what extent this conflict between religious rules and the demands for adult responsibility still contributes to the development of incompetence and diminished self-reliance in adults.

Not only do some biblical rules foster dependency, but they also provide the groundwork for using lack of foresight and incompetence as weapons to coerce others to take care of one's needs. We may recall in this connection that the this-worldly uselessness of the clergy has been rationalized and made possible by the expectation that it is the parishioner's duty to support them. Only in ancient Jewish tradition was this not true. The rabbi had to have a trade so that he would not be forced to accept money for teaching the law of God.

It is implicit in the biblical rules of helplessness that the disabled may regard their weakened status as *prima facie* evidence of merit, which must be rewarded by the appropriate theological, medical, or psychiatric treatment. In the hysterical transaction, disability is used as a coercive tactic to force others to provide for one's needs. It is as if the patient were saying: 'You have told me to be disabled – that is, to act stupid, weak, fearful, etc. You have promised that you would then take care of me, love me, etc. Here I am, acting just as you have told me – it is your turn now to fulfil your promise!' Much of psychoanalytic psychotherapy may revolve around the theme of uncovering exactly who taught the patient to behave in this way, and why he listened to such teachings. It may then be discovered that religion, society, and parents have conspired, so to speak, to uphold and promote this style of behaviour, even though it is so singularly ill-suited to the requirements of our present social conditions.[2]

A Few Historical Comments

As emphasized above, the beliefs and practices of Christianity are best suited for slaves; this is hardly surprising when we recall the oppressed milieu in which this creed emerged.

[2] The rules whereby rewards are offered for *negative possessions* – for example, for *not having* wisdom, foresight, happiness, etc. – pervade the whole of the Christian ethic. Being poor is praised in Matthew 19:23–30; being hungry in Luke 6:20–26; being emasculated in Matthew 19:12. The last mentioned might be worth quoting, because the state of being unsexed, extolled in this passage, will be important for us also in Chapter 10. The relevant lines are: 'For there are some eunuchs, which were so born from *their* mother's womb: and there are some eunuchs, which were made eunuchs of men: and there be eunuchs, which have made themselves eunuchs for the kingdom of heaven's sake.'

Man's emasculation is here codified as one of the ways of courting God's love. The themes of self-castration and impotence – or, more generally, lust and its vicissitudes – are the *leitmotifs* of (1) large parts of the Bible, (2) witchcraft, witch-hunts, and documents dealing with witches, e.g. the *Malleus Maleficarum* (Krämer and Sprenger, 1486), and (3) the early theory of psychoanalysis.

The ethics and psychology of oppression must be contrasted with the ethics and psychology of democracy and equality. Lincoln (1858) said: 'As I would not be a slave, so I would not be a master. This expresses my idea of democracy. Whatever differs from this, to the extent of the difference, is not democracy.' If we define a free, self-governing, democratic man as did Abraham Lincoln – that is, as one who rejects the roles of both master and slave – then we have the picture of a man into whose scheme of life the biblical rules fit poorly or not at all.

Taken in their entirety and removed from any particular historical context, the following generalization may be made concerning biblical rules: *although some of the rules aim at mitigation of oppression, the over-all thesis nevertheless fosters the same oppressive spirit from which these rules arose and with which their creators must inevitably have been imbued.* Since oppressed and oppressor form a functional pair, their psychology – that is, their respective orientations to human relationships – tend to be similar. This is also fostered by the basic human tendency for persons to identify with those with whom they interact. Hence, each slave is a potential master and each master a potential slave. This must be emphasized because it is inaccurate and misleading to contrast the psychology of the oppressed with the psychology of the oppressor. Instead, the common orientation of each should be contrasted with the psychology of the person who feels equal to his fellow man.

Almost always, the simplest way for the oppressed to ameliorate their lot is by changing the rules of the game of life, making new rules more favourable to themselves. In other words, in early Christianity an attempt was made to change the rules and to recruit people to espouse the new rules.

Warfare and forceful subjugation are the traditional methods for enforcing new rules. These methods, however, are useful only for the strong. The weak must rely on more subtle techniques of persuasion. The early versus the later histories of many groups – Christianity and psychoanalysis among them – illustrate this principle (Burckhardt, 1868–71). When Christianity arose, it and its supporters were weak, in the sense that they possessed little or no social or political power. Hence, they had to depend on non-coercive methods to spread their views. Later, after their followers had gained considerable power (social, political, military), they did not hesitate to adopt coercive measures (the Crusades and the Inquisition).

Rule-changing was, in my opinion, one of the most significant features of early Christianity. In substituting new rules for old, Jesus was following in the footsteps of Moses (or perhaps of the Jews generally). The essence of the new rules lay in reversing the old rules, so that 'the first shall be last, and the last shall be first' (Matthew 19:30, 20:16; Mark 10:31; Luke 13:30).

The historical prototype of the rule-reversals advocated by Jesus was originated by Moses (or the Jews). Dissatisfied with their real-life situation, the Jews apparently seized upon the inspired idea that, although they were having a poor time of it in their social relations, they were, in fact, God's Chosen People. Now, to be a chosen or preferred person implies that something especially good will happen to one, even if it is only to receive the love of an unseen God. It is undeniable that, from the psychosocial point of view, this is a most useful manoeuvre. It helps to restore the believer's dangerously weakened self-esteem. In this way he may manage to rise above the degraded position of the oppressed slave and gain a more dignified human stature.

However useful this manoeuvre might have been, its general availability was seriously hampered by the fact that Judaism was not a proselytizing religion. In some respects the Jews imitated the slaveholder group, in that they formed what was essentially a new exclusive club.

Resting on this historical base, Jesus introduced the spirit of democracy into the business of emancipation from slavery. Social status based on personal accomplishment rather than on parentage characterizes modern democratic social organizations. Early Christianity represents a forerunner of this contemporary trend – for it was Jesus who stated that the new rules shall apply to all who wish to embrace them. This far-reaching democratization of Judaism must have contributed to the vast social success of Christianity.

By new rules I refer, of course, to some of the rules set forth in the New Testament. The New Testament must not be contrasted with the Old Testament, for the new rules reversed not those of Judaism but rather those of the social order which prevailed at that time. What were these rules? In general, it was an advantage to be a free citizen of Rome and a believer in Roman polytheism; it was also an advantage to be healthy rather than sick, wealthy rather than poor, admired and beloved rather than persecuted and hated, and so forth. The new rules, as set forth by Jesus and Saint Paul, consisted of a radical reversal of these basic principles. It was asserted that henceforth the 'last' shall be 'first' – 'the loser' shall be the 'winner'. Faithful Christians will now be the winners, pagan Romans the losers. Healthy, wealthy, and admired people will be punished, while the sick, poor, and persecuted will be rewarded.

The new rules possess several features that helped to ensure them popularity and success. In the early days of Christianity there were, of course, many more slaves, sick, poor, and unhappy people than free, healthy, and satisfied ones. This remains true even today. Accordingly, while the rules of the earthly game, as practised in Roman society, held out a promise of opportunity to only a few men, the new rules of Christianity held out the promise of bountiful rewards in a life hereafter to many. In this sense, too, Christianity constituted a move towards democracy and populism.

Today we know only too well that a social rule useful and appropriate at one time and for one purpose may be useless and inappropriate at another time and for another purpose. Although biblical rules once had a largely liberating influence, their effect has long since become politically oppressive and psycho-socially inhibiting. Alas, this transformation has characterized the course of most revolutions, the initial phase of liberation being quickly succeeded by a new phase of oppression (Russell, 1954).

The general principle that a liberating rule may, in due time, become another method of oppression, has broad validity for rule-changing manoeuvres of all types. This is the reason why it is so dangerous today wholeheartedly to espouse new social schemes that offer merely another set of new rules. Although, if social life is to continue as a dynamic process tending towards ever-increasing human complexity and self-determination, new rules are constantly needed, vastly more than mere rule-changing is necessary to attain this goal. In addition to exchanging new rules for old, we must be aware of the rationale of the old rules and guard against their persistent effects. One such effect is to form new rules that are covert reaction-formations against the old rules. Christianity, the French Revolution, Marxism, and even psychoanalysis itself – as a revolution in medicine against the so-called organic tradition – all succumbed to the inescapable fate of all revolutions – the setting up of new tyrannies.

The effects of religious teachings on contemporary Western man is still a delicate subject. Psychiatrists, psychologists, and social scientists tend to avoid it. I have tried to reopen this subject by re-examining some of the values and rules of the Judaeo-Christian religions. If we sincerely desire a scientifically respectable psychosocial theory of man, we shall have to pay far more attention to religious – and perhaps even more to professional – rules and values than has been our custom heretofore.

10 Theology, Witchcraft, and Hysteria

Educators, especially those concerned with inculcating religious teachings, have always endeavoured to get hold of their pupils in early childhood. The idea that religious indoctrination during this period will have a lasting effect on the child's personality antedates psychoanalysis by many centuries. Freud reasserted this opinion when he claimed that a person's character is firmly fixed during the first five or six years of life. Although personally I do not share this view, it is undoubtedly true that the rules on which a human being is fed, as it were, in the early years of life, profoundly affect this later behaviour. This is especially true if a person's 'rule diet' in later years does not differ markedly from that of his childhood. It seems to me that a great deal of a person's later education – say, between the ages of six and early adulthood – is often composed of an educational pabulum containing many of the same nonsensical rules he had been fed earlier. If this is indeed the case, we shall be ill advised to draw far-reaching conclusions about the effects of early learning experiences, since these are often reinforced, rather than modified or corrected, by later influences. I refer here specifically to the values and rules inherent in *religious, national, and professional myths, most of which foster the perpetuation of childish games and mutually coercive patterns of human behaviour.*

What I called 'religious, national, and professional myths' are simply games the main purpose of which is to glorify the group to which the individual belongs (or to membership in which he aspires). Such clannish games must be contrasted with games in which all who are capable of adhering to the rules can participate. The rules of the game based on such a supra-religious and supranational morality would seriously conflict with many of our current habits in living. Nevertheless, I firmly believe that the social trend towards worldwide human equality (of rights and obligations, i.e. to participate in all games according to one's abilities) need not be a threat to men. On the contrary, it represents one of the few values worthy of contemporary man's admiration and support.

In our widespread espousal of clannish myths, we tend to overlook their undesirable effects. The currently operating causes of human disharmony are thus constantly de-emphasized, and the pathogenic significance of past events is exaggerated. I do not deny the psychological significance of past events, but only want to emphasize the significance of dominant contemporary ideologies as determinants of human behaviour. In this connection, it is curious that although everyone's past seems to be full of 'pathogenic' occurrences, few persons seriously entertain the possibility that their current behaviour may continue to provide such harmful experiences for themselves, and also for those about them. Perhaps this pushing of 'pathogenic' experiences from the present into the past is one of the strategies that enables contemporary man to behave as badly in his everyday life as he often does.

In this chapter I shall try to show that, today, the notion of mental illness is used chiefly to obscure and explain away problems in personal and social relationships; and that the notion of witchcraft had been used in the same way during the declining Middle Ages. We now deny moral, personal, political, and social controversies by pretending that they are psychiatric problems: in short, by playing the medical game. During the witch-hunts men denied these controversies by pretending that they were theological problems: in short, by playing the religious game. The religious rules of life and their effects on man in the late Middle Ages thus not only illustrate the principles of rule-following behaviour, but also display the belief in witchcraft as a historical precursor of the modern belief in mental illness.

The Medical Theory of Witchcraft

It is often asserted that the medieval women accused of witchcraft actually suffered from what we now *know* to be hysteria. Numerous medical and psychiatric authors advocate such a psychiatric view of witchcraft.

Zilboorg maintained that witches were misdiagnosed mental patients, a view he based largely on his interpretation of Krämer and Sprenger's *Malleus Maleficarum* (1486). It is clear, however, that Zilboorg was determined to prove that witches were mentally sick persons, and that he disregarded all evidence suggesting other interpretations. He ignored the fact that the *Malleus Maleficarum* shows a much greater resemblance to a legal than to a medical document. The ferreting out of witches and the proving of witchcraft were preliminary to *sentencing*. Although Zilboorg (1935) noted that a large part of the *Malleus* dealt with the legal examination and sentencing of witches, he did not draw the logical inference that witches were criminals, or, to put it more neutrally, offenders against the prevailing social (theological) order. On the contrary, he suggested that 'The *Malleus Maleficarum* might, with a little editing, serve as an excellent modern textbook of descriptive clinical psychiatry of the fifteenth century, if the word *witch* were substituted by the word *patient*, and the devil eliminated' (p. 58).

This interpretation must have seemed too sweeping even for Zilboorg, for later on he offered another opinion which partly contradicts this generalization: 'Not all accused of being witches and sorcerers were mentally sick, but almost all mentally sick were considered witches, or sorcerers, or bewitched' (p. 153).

Although Zilboorg (1941) emphasized that medieval man was engaged in playing a game quite different from that we now play, he proceeded to cast Krämer and Sprenger's observations into a medical and psychiatric mould:

This passage from the *Malleus* is perhaps the most significant statement to come out of the fifteenth century. Here, in a concise and succinct paragraph, *two monks brush aside the whole mass of psychiatric knowledge which had been so carefully collected and preserved by almost two thousand years of medical and philosophic investigation*; they brush it aside almost casually and with such stunning simplicity that no room is left for argument. How can one raise objections to the assertion, 'but this is contrary to true faith'? The fusion of insanity, witchcraft and heresy into one concept and the exclusion of even the suspicion that *the problem is a medical one* are now complete. ([Italics added] p. 155)

Farther on, he added:

The belief in the free will of man is here brought to its most terrifying, although most preposterous, conclusion. Man, whatever *he does, even if he succumbs to an illness* which perverts his perceptions, imagination, and intellectual functions, does it of his own free will; he voluntarily bows to the wishes of the Evil One. The devil does not lure and trap man; man chooses to succumb to the devil and he must be held responsible for this free choice. He must be punished; he must be eliminated from the community. ([Italics added] p. 156)

Following Zilboorg, it has become popular for psychiatrists to assume – indeed, to insist – that witches were unfortunate women who 'fell ill' with 'mental illness'. This interpretation must be challenged. The notion that so-called witches were mentally ill people discredits the entire theological world view underlying the belief in witchcraft, and enthrones the concept of mental illness as an explanatory theory of wide scope and unchallenged power.

Zilboorg asserts that the authors of the *Malleus* had brushed aside two thousand years of medical and psychiatric knowledge. But what medical and psychiatric knowledge was there in the fifteenth century that would have been relevant to the problems to which the theologians addressed themselves? Surely, the ideas of Galenic medicine would have been irrelevant. In fact, medieval man possessed no 'medical' knowledge relevant to the problem of witchcraft. Nor was any such knowledge needed, for there was abundant evidence that charges of witchcraft were commonly trumped up for the purpose of eliminating certain people, and that confessions were extorted by means of cruel tortures (Parrinder, 1958). Finally, if the belief in witchcraft was a 'medical mistake' – codifying the mis-diagnosis of hysterics as witches – why was this mistake not made more often prior to the thirteenth century?

To explain witchcraft Zilboorg offered a medical explanation without specifying how it was to be used. To what sort of illness do people said to be 'mentally ill' succumb? Is it to diseases such as paresis or brain tumour? Or is it to problems in living, arising from – or at the very least precipitated by – family and social pressures, conflicting goals, and so forth? None of these questions is raised, much less answered, by the proponents of the medical theory of witchcraft. Zilboorg's interpretation that the imputation of witchcraft signified a fanatical belief in free will is simply false. It contradicts the most obvious fact – namely, that the majority of witches were women, especially old, poor, and socially readily expendable women. Moreover, when people were considered to be possessed by the devil, it was generally not attributed to their free will, but was viewed rather as occurring against their 'better judgement'. Accordingly, the witch-hunters were regarded as the agents of their unfortunate clients – and executing witches was defined as 'therapeutic'. This total-itarian definition of what constitutes 'therapy' and of who is a 'therapist' has persisted to our day with respect to all involun-tary psychiatric interventions (Szasz, 1957d).

The medical theory of witchcraft ignores two obvious social determinants of the belief in witches and its corollary, witch-hunts. Firstly, a preoccupation with God, Jesus, and Christian theology cannot be arbitrarily separated from a belief in bad deities and their cohorts (devils, witches, sorcerers). Secondly, concern with the sexual activities of witches and devils was a counterpart, a mirror-image, of the officially antisexual attitude of the Catholic Church. The torturing and burning of witches must be viewed in the light of medieval man's theological world view according to which the body is weak and sinful, and the only goal worthy of man is the eternal salvation of the soul (Huizinga, 1927). Thus, burning human bodies at the stake was a symbolic act which expressed adherence to the official rules of the game. This dramatic, ritualized affirmation of the faith insured the continued existence of an important social fiction or myth (Vaihinger, 1911). From this point of view, burning witches may be compared to destroying confiscated whisky during prohibition. Both acts gave official recognition to a rule which few people followed in their actual conduct. During the Middle Ages sexual conduct was, actually, exceedingly promis-cuous if measured by our current standards (Lewinsohn, 1958).

In both instances, then, the law expressed high ethical ideals to which most people had no intention to adhere. Their goal became, instead, to evade the laws, to appear as if they were law-abiding, and to make sure that there were appropriate others who were caught and punished. For this *scapegoats* were needed. In situations of this sort, it is the scapegoat's social function to play the role of the person who violates (or is said to violate) the rules, is caught, and is duly punished (Nadel, 1954, pp. 205–6). We might thus view bootleggers and the entire class of so-called organized gangsters – all of whom came into being while prohibition was the law of the land in the United States – as the scapegoats who were sacrificed at the altar of the false god of abstinence. The greater the actual discrepancy between prescribed rules of conduct and actual social behaviour, the greater the need for scapegoat-sacrifices as a means of maintaining the social myth that man lives according to his officially declared ethical beliefs.

The Scapegoat Theory of Witchcraft

I submit that witchcraft represents the expression of a particular method by means of which men have sought to explain and master various ills of nature. Unable to admit ignorance and helplessness, yet equally unable to achieve scientific understanding and mastery of diverse physical, biological, and social problems, men have sought refuge in scapegoat explanations. The specific identities of the scapegoats are legion: lepers, witches, women, Jews, Negroes, the mentally ill, and so forth. All scapegoat theories postulate that if only the offending person, race, illness, or what-not could be dominated, subjugated, mastered, or eliminated, all manner of problems would be solved.

While medical men subscribe enthusiastically to the idea that witches were hysterical women who had been mis-diagnosed, social scientists lean towards the view that they were society's scapegoats (Parrinder, 1958). I am in substantial agreement with this latter interpretation, and shall try to show exactly in what ways the scapegoat theory is superior to the medical one. In addition, I shall argue that not only is it misleading to consider witches mis-diagnosed hysterics, but it is also misleading to regard people currently 'ill' with hysteria (or other mental illnesses) as belonging in the same category as those ill with bodily ailments.

With respect to the scapegoat theory of witchcraft, we might raise the following questions: Who were considered to be witches? How were they tried and who profited from their conviction? What did those people who did not believe in the reality of witches think of witchcraft? Did they think that witches were ill? Or did they believe that the problem was not one of witchcraft at all, but that it was a matter of trumped-up charges? In discussing these questions, I shall try to develop the similarities between the medieval belief in witchcraft and the contemporary belief in mental illness; and I shall try to show that both are false explanations that conceal certain difficult moral problems. Moreover, both serve the interests of a special group – the one, the interests of the clergy, the other those of the medical profession. Finally, both fulfil their function by sacrificing a special group of persons on the altar of social expedience: in the Middle Ages the scapegoats were the witches; today, they are the involuntary mental patients and the mentally ill generally.

In comparing witchcraft with mental illness it is important to bear in mind that the traditional concept of illness rests on the simple facts of pain, suffering, and disability. Hence the sufferer, the patient himself, first considers himself ill, and is then usually so considered by others. In sociological terms (Parsons, 1952), *the sick role in medicine is typically self-defined*.

The traditional concept of mental illness, or insanity, rests on precisely the opposite definitions. The alleged sufferer (especially the 'psychotic') considers himself neither sick nor disabled; but others insist that he is both! The role of mental patient is thus often imposed on persons against their will. In short, *the sick role in psychiatry is typically other-defined*.

This distinction between being a patient by one's own definition or choice or being so defined against one's will is all-important: the mentally sick role is self-defined usually in the hope and expectation that this manoeuvre will help to secure certain types of help, for example private psychotherapy; in contrast, when this role is imposed on a person against his will, the manoeuvre serves the interests of those who define him as mentally ill.

How did people ascertain, during the Middle Ages, that someone was a witch? Of course, individuals rarely 'discovered' that *they themselves* were witches. Rather, some persons or groups claimed – and it was subsequently ascertained, by the methods then prescribed – that *someone else* was a witch. In other words, the witch role was characteristically other-defined. The role of witch was thus similar to the contemporary role of involuntary mental patient.

Most people accused of witchcraft were women. The word 'witch' implies 'woman', as did the word 'hysteric'. Janet and Freud, it will be remembered, were pioneers in asserting that there were 'male hysterics'.[1] In this respect, the parallels between being a witch and being a hysteric are striking. According to Parrinder (1958), out of two hundred convicted witches in England, only fifteen were men (p. 54). He interpreted this as a sign that women were a persecuted minority in a world ruled by men.

In addition to the high incidence of women, most persons accused of witchcraft were members of the lower classes. They were poor, stupid, socially helpless, and often old and feeble. Making a 'diagnosis' of witchcraft then – much as calling someone mentally ill today – was an insult and an accusation. Obviously, it is safer to accuse socially unimportant persons than those who are socially prominent. When highly placed persons were accused of witchcraft, as happened occasionally, it was safer as well as more effective if the charge was made by large groups, as for instance a whole nunnery, rather than by a single person. Then, as now, there was safety in numbers – the

[1] The discovery of 'male hysteria', like Charcot's conversion of malingerers to hysterics (see Chapter 1), was another step in the *democratization of misery*. Freud (1932) was apparently more eager to acknowledge equality between the sexes in regard to suffering (i.e. susceptibility to 'neurosis') than in regard to potentialities for creative performance! His assertion that men, too, may suffer from hysteria must be contrasted with his equally firm conviction that women were incapable of the same types of work, 'sublimations', and 'mental development' as men.

assumption being that if many people claimed something, it had to be true! Nevertheless, the educated and the well-to-do could better protect themselves from the danger of being branded witches and being 'treated' for it (by burning at the stake), much as well-informed and wealthy persons today have less difficulty avoiding being diagnosed 'mentally ill' against their will. They are thus able to avoid commitment, loss of civil liberties, and 'treatment' by means of electric shocks, lobotomies, and the like – the fate of those less fortunate.

Actually, the medieval inquisitors themselves were impressed by the discrepancy between the patently feeble and harmless character of the women accused of witchcraft and their allegedly diabolical and potent actions. Parrinder (1958) commented:

The explanation was given that their evil deeds had been performed by the help of the devil, but that, like the deceiver he is, he had abandoned his disciples in their moment of need ... This was very convenient for the inquisitors, for it meant that they could handle these dangerous women without risk to themselves. (p. 58)

Although Parrinder called these antifeminine attitudes, beliefs, and actions 'ridiculous', this should not divert our attention from the fact that essentially similar attitudes were prevalent in Europe well into the twentieth century. In fact, such prejudices are by no means extinct today, even in so-called civilized countries. In the economically underdeveloped areas of the world, the systematic oppression and exploitation of women – much like slavery and the exploitation of alien races – remain the dominant customs and rules of life.

While these historical and cultural considerations are of momentous importance in so far as any progress towards an internationally meaningful science of human behaviour is contemplated, what is even more significant, especially in relation to hysteria, is the cultural attitude towards women in Central Europe at the turn of the century. This was the time and place of the origin of psychoanalysis, and, through it, of the entire body of what is now known as 'dynamic psychiatry'. That the status of women in that social situation was still one of profound oppression, while well known, is easily forgotten or relegated to a position of unimportance. Generally, women were then economically dependent on their parents or spouses, had few educational and occupational opportunities, and were regarded – perhaps not quite explicitly – as the mere bearers of uteri. Their 'proper' role and function were marriage and motherhood. Accordingly, they were considered biologically inferior to men in regard to such traits as intellectual ability and finer ethical feelings. Some of Freud's opinions about women were not unlike those of Krämer and Sprenger.

The following is typical of Freud's (1932) views on what he called 'the psychology of women':

It must be admitted that women have but little sense of justice, and this is no doubt connected with the preponderance of envy in their mental life; for the demands of justice *are* a modification of envy; they lay down the conditions under which one is willing to part with it. We also say of women that their *social interests are weaker* than those of men, and that their capacity for the *sublimation of their instincts is less*. ([Italics added] p. 183)

I cite this opinion of Freud's about women not so much to criticize it – that has been adequately done by others (A. Adler, 1907–37; Horney, 1939; Fromm, 1959) – but to emphasize the significance of scapegoating in the phenomena called witchcraft, hysteria, and mental illness.

The belief in witches, devils, and their cohorts was, of course, more than just a matter of metaphysics or theological theory. It affected public behaviour – most glaringly in the form of witch-hunts and witch-trials. In a way, these were the opposites or mirror images of saintly miracles. Alleged acts of witchcraft or miracle-working could be officially recognized only after they had been passed on and approved as valid by the holders of appropriate social power – in this case, the high-ranking clergy of the Roman Catholic church. The genuineness of acts of witchcraft, sorcery, and so forth were established by what was basically a legal procedure, set in a theological context. Hence the expression 'witch-trials'. Obviously, a trial is neither a medical nor a scientific affair.

The distinction between legal and scientific disputes was recognized by medieval man, no less than by the ancients. Yet, this important distinction was obscured by the medical theory of hysteria. Legal contests serve to settle disputes of conflicting interests. Medical procedures serve to settle the nature of the patient's illness and the measures that might restore him to health. In such a situation there are no obvious conflicts of interest between opposing parties. The patient is ill and wants to recover; his family and society also want him to recover; so does his physician.

The situation is different in a legal dispute where the problem is a conflict of interests between two or more parties. What is good ('therapeutic') for one party, is likely to be bad ('noxious') for the other. Instead of a situation of co-operation between patient and physician, we have one of conciliation between two contending parties, with the judge serving as arbitrator of the dispute.

In European witch-trials it was customary for the judge to receive a portion of the convicted heretic's worldly possessions (Parrinder, 1958, p. 79). Today, we take it for granted that, in free societies, the judge is impartial. His task is to uphold the law. Hence he must occupy a position outside the socio-economic interests of the litigants. While all this may seem dreadfully obvious, it needs to be said because, even today, the impartiality of the judge towards the litigants is often an unrealized ideal. In totalitarian countries, for example, so-called crimes against the state fall in the same class as witch-trials: the judge is an employee of one of the contesting parties. Even in free societies, in crimes violating cardinal moral and social beliefs – such as treason or subversion – judicial impartiality is often thrown to the wind – and we have 'political justice'. This is why 'political criminals' may become 'revolutionary heroes', and, should the revolution fail, revert once more to the status of 'criminals'.

In witch-trials the conflict was officially defined as between the accused and God, or between the accused and the Catholic (later Protestant) Church, as God's earthly representative. There was no attempt to make this an even match. The distribution of power between accuser and accused mirrored the relations between king and serf – one had all the power and the other none of it. Once again we encounter the theme of domination and submission. Significantly, only in England – where, beginning in the thirteenth century with the granting of the Magna Charta, there gradually developed an appreciation of the rights and dignities of those less powerful than the king – was the fury of witch-hunting mitigated by legal safeguards and social sensibilities.

Behind the ostensible conflict of the witch-trial lay the usual conflicts of social class, values, and human relationships. Furthermore, there was strife within the Catholic Church itself which later became accentuated by the antagonisms between Catholics and Protestants. It was in this context, then, that witches and sorcerers, recruited from the ranks of the poor and oppressed, played the role of scapegoats. They thus fulfilled the socially useful function of acting as social tranquillizers (Szasz, 1960c). By participating in an important public drama, they contributed to the stability of the existing social order.

Games of Life: Theological and Medical

Life in the Middle Ages was a colossal religious game. The dominant value was salvation in a life hereafter (Huizinga, 1927). Gallinek (1942), emphasizing that 'to divorce medieval hysteria from its time and place is not possible' (p. 42), observed:

It was the aim of man to leave all things worldly as far behind as possible, and already during lifetime to approach the kingdom of heaven. The aim was salvation. Salvation was the Christian master motive. The ideal man of the Middle Ages was free of all fear because he was sure of salvation, certain of eternal bliss. He was the saint, and the saint, not the knight nor the troubadour, is the veritable ideal of the Middle Ages. (p. 47)

However, if sainthood and salvation formed one part of the Christian game of life, witchcraft and damnation formed another. The two belong together in a single system of beliefs and rules, just as, say, military decorations for bravery and punishments for desertion belong together. Positive and negative sanctions, or rewards and penalties, form a complementary pair and share equally in giving form and substance to the game. A game is composed of the totality of its rules. If any of the rules is changed, the game itself is changed. It is important to keep this clearly in mind to avoid the sentimental belief that the essential identity of a game may be preserved by retaining only its desirable features (rewards), and eliminating all that is undesirable (penalties).

On the contrary, if preservation of the game – that is, maintenance of the social (religious) *status quo* – is desired, this can be best achieved by enthusiastically playing the game as it is. Thus, searching for and finding witches constituted an important manoeuvre for playing the religious game of life, much as looking for and finding mental illness is a convenient tactic for keeping the contemporary medical-therapeutic game alive and vigorous. The extent to which belief in and preoccupation with witchcraft constituted a part of the theological game of life may be gleaned from Parrinder's (1958) description of 'Pacts with the Devil' (p. 68).

It is significant that the criteria for 'diagnosing' witchcraft and heresy were of the same type as the criteria for establishing the possession of genuine belief. Both were inferred from what the person *said*. I wish to emphasize the great importance that was attributed, at that time, to what people verbalized about their beliefs, feelings, and experiences. Claims of devotion to God or of having seen the Holy Virgin were thus elevated to a rank even higher than deeds. Honest service and decent behaviour counted for naught, while extravagant claims were sometimes magnificently rewarded.

Similar methods were used to establish a person's 'badness'. Observable occurrences were de-emphasized in favour of self-revelations obtained, if necessary, under torture. All this took place, moreover, in a social setting in which brutal behaviour – especially on the part of noblemen towards serfs, men towards women, adults towards children – was an everyday matter. Its very ubiquity must have dulled men's sensibilities and turned their attention from it. It is not easy to remain interested in what is commonplace – such as man's everyday brutality vis-à-vis his fellow-man. Oh, but the dastardly behaviour of persons in the grips of the devil ... That was another, more interesting matter! Since this could not be directly observed, the 'diagnosticians' of sorcery and witchcraft had to rely heavily on verbal communications. These were of two kinds: first, accusations against persons concerning the commission of evil deeds or peculiar acts, and second, confessions of misdeeds.

Let us now examine the values of a social system that encourages the 'diagnosis' of hysteria. Clearly, one of the principal values of our culture is science. Medicine, as a part of science, enters this value system. The notions of health, illness, and treatment are thus the cornerstones of an all-embracing modern medical-therapeutic world view (Szasz, 1958b).

In speaking of science as a widely shared social value, I do not refer to any particular scientific method, nor have I in mind such things as the search for 'truth', 'understanding', or 'explanation'. I refer rather to science as an institutional force, similar to organized theology in the past. It is to this aspect of 'science', sometimes called 'scientism', that increasing numbers of people turn in their search for practical guidance in living. According to this scheme of values, one of the most important things for man to achieve is to have a strong and healthy body – a wish that is the true heir to medieval man's wish for a virtuous soul. A healthy body is regarded as useful not, it is true, for salvation, but for comfort, sex appeal, happiness, and a long life. Great efforts and vast sums are expended in pursuit of this goal of having a healthy – and this has of late included an *attractive* – body. Finally, having a healthy 'mind' has been added to this value-scheme by regarding the 'mind' as if it were simply another part of the human organism. In this view, the human being is endowed with a skeletal system, digestive system, circulatory system, nervous system, etc. – *and* a 'mind'. Or, as the Romans had put it, *Mens sana in corpora sano*: 'In a healthy body, a healthy mind.' Strangely enough, much of modern psychiatry has been devoted to this ancient proposition. Psychiatrists who search for biological (genetic, biochemical, etc.) abnormalities as the causes of 'mental illness' are, whether they know it or not, committed to this frame of reference and its covert values.

Even if we do not believe in the reducibility of psychiatry to biochemistry, the notion of mental illness implies, firstly, that mental health is a 'good thing'; and secondly, that there are certain criteria according to which mental health and illness can be diagnosed. In the name of this value, then, the same sorts of actions may be justified as were justified by medieval man marching under the banner of God and Christ. What are some of these actions?

Those who are considered especially strong and healthy – or who contribute to these values – are rewarded. The athletes, the beauty queens, and the movie stars are the modern-day 'saints' – and the cosmetics manufacturers, doctors, psychiatrists, and so forth, their assistants. They are honoured, admired, and rewarded. All this is well known and should occasion little surprise. Who are the people who fall in the class of the witches and sorcerers: the people persecuted and victimized in the name of 'health' and 'happiness'? They are legion. In their front ranks are the mentally ill, and especially those who are so defined by others rather than by themselves. The involuntarily hospitalized mentally ill are regarded as 'bad' and efforts are made to make them 'better'. Words like 'good' and 'bad' are used here in accordance with the value system in force. Though this is an ostensibly medical system of values, it is none the less an ethical scheme. In addition to the mentally ill, elderly persons and people who are ugly or deformed find themselves in a class analogous to the now defunct category of witches and sorcerers.

The reason why individuals displaying such characteristics are considered 'bad' is inherent in the rules of the medical game. Just as witchcraft was an inverted theological game, so much of general psychiatry – especially the so-called care of the involuntary mental patient – is a kind of inverted medical game. The rules of the medical game define health – which includes such things as a well-functioning body and happiness – as a positive value. Illness thus becomes the opposite – that is, an ill-functioning body and unhappiness or depression. Hysteria, as we have seen, is a dramatized representation of the message: 'My body is not functioning well.' And the mental illness called 'depression' is a dramatization of the proposition: 'I am unhappy.'

In so far as people adhere to the ethics of the medical game, sick patients will, at least to some extent, be disliked. This tends to be mitigated by the sick person's submission to those who attempt to make him well and by his own efforts to recover. In many ways, however, patients with hysteria, and with mental illnesses generally, do not make 'appropriate' efforts to get well. To that extent they forfeit the ordinary person's and the physician's disposition to behave kindly towards them and invite more or less thinly disguised hostility. In this framework of medical ethics, the patient deserves kindness only in so far as he is potentially healthy. This is similar to the medieval religious ethic according to which the witch or the heretic was worthy of human attention only in so far as he was a potential 'true believer'. In the one case, man is accepted as human – and thus deserving of humane treatment – only because he might be healthy; in the other, only because he might be a good Christian. Thus, neither sickness nor religious disbelief were given the kind of humane recognition they deserved.

It is easy, of course, to be sceptical of a belief that no longer commands wide adherence. Hence, people find it easy now to doubt religion. But our present world view is medical, not religious. And, indeed, people find it anything but easy to doubt the pronouncements of medicine, and especially of psychiatry. This is why the idea that illness, and particularly mental illness, should be an acceptable, legitimate way of life seems as absurd to most people today as the idea that heresy should have been an acceptable, legitimate way of life would have seemed to the men of the Middle Ages.

PART IV
Game-model Analysis of Behaviour

11 The Game-playing Model of Human Behaviour

George H. Mead on Human Actions as Games

Much of what I have said so far has utilized a game model of human behaviour, first clearly formulated by George Herbert Mead (1934). His thesis was that mind and self are generated in a social process and that linguistic communication is the single most important feature responsible for the differences between the behaviour of animals and men.

Mead considered games as paradigmatic of social situations. Accordingly, they were of the greatest significance in his theory of human behaviour which regarded man as essentially a role-taking animal. Playing a game presupposes that each player is able to take the role of all the other players. Mead also emphasized that game rules are of great interest to children and are crucial to the social development of the human being.

The social situation in which a person lives constitutes the team on which he plays and is, therefore, of the utmost importance in determining *who he is* and *how he acts*. Man's so-called instinctual needs are actually shaped – and this may include inhibiting, fostering, or even creating 'needs' – by the social game prevalent in his milieu. The view of a dual, biosocial determination of behaviour has become integrated into psychoanalytic theory through increasing emphasis on ego-psychology and object relationships. Useful as these modifications of classical psychoanalytic theory have been, explanations in terms of ego-functions are not as adequate for either theory or therapy as those couched in terms of rules, roles, and games.

In this connection, let us briefly consider a problem that illuminates the connections between psychoanalysis and game theory (in the sense used here) – namely, the problem of primary and secondary gains. In psychoanalysis, gains derived from playing a game profitably – say, by being protectively treated for an hysterical illness – are regarded as secondary. As the term betrays, these gains are considered less significant as reasons, or motives, for the behaviour in question than primary gains, which are derived from the gratifications of unconscious instinctual needs.

If we reinterpret these phenomena in terms of a consistently game-playing model of behaviour, there will be no need to distinguish between primary and secondary gains. The correlative necessity to estimate the relative significance of physiological needs and dammed-up impulses on the one hand and of social and interpersonal factors on the other also disappears. Since needs and impulses cannot be said to exist in human social life without specified rules for dealing with them, instinctual needs cannot be considered solely in terms of biological rules, but must also be viewed in terms of their psychosocial significance – that is, as parts of the game.

It follows that what we call 'hysteria' or 'mental illness' can be properly understood only in the context of a specified social setting. While diseases such as syphilis and tuberculosis are in the nature of *events* and hence can be described without taking cognizance of how men conduct themselves in their social affairs, hysteria, and all other so-called mental illnesses are in the nature of *actions*. They are thus *made to happen* by sentient intelligent human beings and can be understood best, in my opinion, in the framework of games. Mental illnesses thus differ fundamentally from bodily diseases, and resemble, rather, certain moves or tactics in playing games.

Jean Piaget on the Development of Games

I have used the notion of games so far as if it were familiar to most people. I think this is justified as everyone knows how to play some games. Accordingly, games serve admirably as models for the clarification of other, less well-understood, social-psychological phenomena. Yet the ability to follow rules, play games, and construct new games is a faculty not equally shared by all persons. It will thus be helpful to consider the child's development in regard to his ability to play games.

Piaget (1928, 1932, 1951), who has carefully studied the evolution of games during childhood, suggested that moral behaviour be viewed as a type of rule-following: 'All morality consists in a system of rules, and the essence of all morality is to be sought for in the respect which the individual acquires for these rules' (1932, p. 1). Piaget thus equated the nature of morality, or ethical feeling and conduct, with the individual's attitude towards and practice of various rules. This perspective provides a rational basis for the analysis of moral schemes as games, and of moral behaviour as the players' actual conduct.

In his studies of game rules, Piaget distinguished two distinct features of rule-following behaviour: one, the practice of rules, that is, the ways in which children of different ages apply rules; the other, the consciousness of rules, that is, self-reflection about the rules and role-taking behaviour. He noted that children of different ages have different ideas concerning the character of the game rules: younger children regard them as obligatory, externally imposed, and 'sacred', whereas older children learn to regard rules as socially defined and, in a sense, self-imposed. Piaget thus traced rule-following and game-playing behaviour from early childhood stages of egocentrism, imitation, and heteronomy to the later (mature) stage of co-operation, rational rule-following, and autonomy (pp. 86–95). Since for our purpose the details of the development of rule-following behaviour are not relevant, only a brief summary of Piaget's scheme will be presented.

Piaget distinguished four stages in the practice or *application of rules*. The earliest stage is characterized by the automatic imitation by the pre-verbal child of certain behaviour-patterns he observes in others. Piaget called these motor rules, which later become habits. The second stage begins some time after the second year of life, 'when the child receives from the outside the example of codified rules' (p. 16). His play during this phase is purely egocentric: he plays in the presence of others, but not with them. This type of rule-application is characterized by a combination of imitation[1] of others with an idiosyncratic use

[1] Piaget (1932) characterized this stage as consisting of the 'imitation of seniors with egocentrism' (p. 41). It is no accident that the notion of imitation recurs here once again. Using imitation as a key concept, denoting by it pro-

of the examples received. For example, everyone can win at once. This stage usually ends at about the age of seven or eight years.

During the third stage, designated as the stage of incipient co-operation, children 'begin to concern themselves with the question of mutual control and of the unification of rules' (p. 17). Nevertheless, play remains relatively idiosyncratic. When during this period children are questioned about the rules of the game in which they are engaged, they often give entirely contradictory accounts of them. The fourth stage appears between the ages of eleven and twelve years and is characterized by the codification of rules. The rules of the game are now well understood; there is a correspondingly high degree of consensus among children about what they are. The game rules are now explicit, public, and conventional.

This scheme must be supplemented by the development of the *consciousness of rules* – that is, the person's experience in regard to the origin and nature of the rules, and especially his feeling and conception about how they obligate him to obey the rules. Piaget (1932) described three stages in the development of rule-consciousness. During the first stage 'rules are not yet coercive in character, either because they are purely motor, or else (at the beginning of the egocentric stage) because they are received, as it were, unconsciously, and as interesting examples rather than as obligatory realities' (p. 18). During the second stage, which begins at about the age of five years, rules are regarded as sacred and untouchable. Games composed of such rules are called heteronomous. The rules emanate from the adults and are experienced as lasting for ever: 'Every suggested alteration strikes the child as a transgression' (p. 18). The third and final stage begins when the child regards rules as acquiring their obligatory character from mutual consent. Such rules must be obeyed because loyalty to the group, or to the game, demands it. Undesirable rules, however, can be altered. It is this attitude

---

cesses of individual development on the one hand and social concepts (such as rules, roles, and games) on the other, I shall try to show that an analysis of hysteria in terms of the game model and the interpretations offered previously in terms of communication and rule-following converge to form a single theory.

towards games that we usually associate with and expect of an adult in a free society. Such a person is expected to know and feel that just as the rules of a game are man-made, so are the laws of a nation. This may be contrasted with the rules of the game of a theocratic society, in which the citizen is expected to believe that the laws are God-given. So-called autonomous games, in contrast to heteronomous ones, can be played only by individuals who have reached the last stages in the foregoing developmental schemes.

The evolution of the child's concept of games and rules parallels the development of his intelligence. The ability to distinguish biological from social rules thus depends on a certain degree of intellectual and moral development. This makes it readily understandable why it is during adolescence that children begin to have doubts concerning the rationality of biblical rules. It seems to me, therefore, that much of what has been labelled 'adolescent rebelliousness' may be attributed to the fact that it is only at this time that children have enough sense to be able intelligently to scrutinize parental, religious, and social demands as systems of rules. The Bible lends itself especially well to criticism by the developing logical sense of the adolescent, for in it biological and social rules are often un-differentiated, or deliberately confused. In Piaget's terms, all rules are treated as if they were parts of heteronomous games. This type of game fits best into the world of a less than ten-year-old child.

Since children, especially very young children, are completely dependent on their parents, their relative inability to compre-hend other than externally imposed, coercive rules is not surprising. In the same way, to the extent that adults depend, or are made to depend, on others rather than on themselves, their game-playing attitudes will approximate to those of children.

Personality Development and Moral Values

According to Piaget, the evolution of children's games proceeds from heteronomy to autonomy. In terms of interpersonal processes aimed at mastery, this corresponds to a movement from coercion towards self-help and reciprocal co-operation among equals. Although Piaget described these psychological and social phenomena with great fidelity, I believe that he did not emphasize enough the ethical dimensions implicit in them. For what Piaget described is, I think, mainly the kind of development which some members of the middle and upper classes of contemporary Western nations want for their own children, or for themselves. Autonomy, integrity, and mutually respectful co-operation are the principal values and developmental goals towards which this process of socialization aims. But are these the values for which the lower classes strive or which some of the organized religions promote? It does not seem to me that they are. Lower-class persons – that is, men and women with little education, and perhaps in dire economic straits – tend to seek power and domination rather than equality. Of course, this striving for power, domination, and exploitation of others is not limited to members of any particular social class.

Domination–Submission versus Equality and Reciprocity

The fundamental human conflict between domination–submission and equality may be seen, in various forms, in virtually all human affairs. The French revolution, for example, was waged in the names of *Liberté, égalité, et fraternité*. Two of these values – equality and fraternity – imply co-operation rather than oppression. Yet the co-operative value-ideals of the philosophers who provided the original impetus for the revolution soon gave way to the pragmatically held values of the masses. These values, in turn, did not differ greatly from the values by which the oppressed masses had been ruled by sovereign royalty. Power, coercion, and oppression soon replaced equality, fraternity, and co-operation.

In the next major European revolution, the moral values of the lower classes received a more unconcealed expression. The Marxist revolution promised a *dictatorship* of the proletariat: the oppressed shall become the oppressors! This was rather similar to the scriptural programme which promised that 'the last shall be the first'. The main difference between the two lay in their respective means of implementation.

'Natural Superiority' versus Postnatal Experience

I do not believe in the 'natural' superiority or inferiority of any group of human beings. And I believe that the effects of education, broadly conceived, are still one of the most underestimated phenomena in the modern world. Accordingly, I reject the traditional belief in the natural superiority of men – or of white men, 'civilized' men, etc. – as well as the easily predictable reaction-formation to it which has proclaimed the 'natural superiority' of women (Montagu, 1953). This does not mean that I do not consider well-educated men to be vastly different from uneducated ones. Since uneducated men cannot compete on equal footing in the game of life with their better educated brothers, they tend to become chronic losers. Players who always lose cannot be expected to harbour affectionate feelings towards either the game or their opponents.

Personality as a Normative Psychosocial Conception

The conception of a distinctive 'human' or well-functioning personality is rooted in psychosocial and ethical criteria. It is not biologically given, nor are biological determinants especially significant for it. I do not deny, of course, that man is an animal with a genetically determined biological equipment which sets the upper and lower limits within which he must function. I accept the limits, or the general range, and focus on the development of specific patterns of operation within them. Hence, I eschew biological considerations as explanations, and instead try to construct a consistently moral and psychosocial explanatory scheme.

Clearly, different societies exhibit different values. And even within a single society, especially if it is composed of many individuals, adults and growing children have certain choices about which values to teach and which to accept or reject. In contemporary Western societies, the principal alternatives are between autonomy and heteronomy – or between 'risky' freedom and 'secure' slavery. (This is an oversimplification which I offer mainly for the purpose of further orientation.)

Piaget (1932) wrote:

> *In our societies the child, as he grows up, frees himself more and more from adult authority; whereas in the lower grades of civilization puberty marks the beginning of an increasingly marked subjection of the individual to the elders and to the traditions of his tribe.* And this is why collective responsibility seems to us to be missing from the moral make-up of the child, whereas it is a notion that is fundamental in the code of primitive ethics. ([Italics added] p. 250)

We have seen (Chapter 10), however, that encouragement to strive towards adult integrity by emancipation from the unilateral authority of others is not the only active moral incentive in our society. Piaget himself commented on some of the forces that foster coercive, power-dependent, heteronomous behaviour:

> It looks as though, in many ways, *the adult did everything in his power to encourage the child to persevere in its specific tendencies, and to do so precisely in so far as these tendencies stand in the way of social development.* Whereas, given sufficient liberty of action, the child will spontaneously emerge from his egocentrism and tend with his whole being towards co-operation, *the adult most of the time acts in such a way as to strengthen egocentrism in its double aspect, intellectual and moral.* ([Italics added] p. 188)

Although I agree with Piaget that some types of adult behaviour foster the child's egocentrism, I doubt that the child would emerge from this stage and move towards autonomy spontaneously. Reciprocity and autonomy are complex values concerning human relationships and must also be taught. Naturally, they cannot be taught coercively, but must be practised and be made examples for the child to emulate.

Piaget singled out the adult's coercive or autocratic attitude towards the child as a cause for his persistent subservience in later life. Such infantilizing-oppressive influences are, of course, not limited to the family situation. On the contrary, they are ubiquitous and may be found in educational, religious, medical and other settings. I noted previously that egocentrism, rather than co-operation and autonomy, is fostered by certain religious teachings. The means by which submission, dependency, and infantilism are fostered in medicine and psychiatry have often been discussed (e.g. Meerloo, 1955; Szasz and Hollender, 1956). Although important for all of medicine, this matter is especially important for psychiatry, because psychiatric patients are particularly uncertain of their social and moral behaviour. Since social conduct has a more specific as well as a more powerful impact on one's sense of identity than do physiological processes, restrictions on it have more far-reaching psychological effects. This is another way of saying that interpersonally, politically, or socially imposed limitations on freedom are often more crippling than those imposed by physical disability.

It has long been known that bodily disability predisposes to hysterical illness. Freud (Breuer and Freud, 1893–5, p. 40) spoke of this as 'somatic compliance' and Ferenczi (1916–17) as 'pathoneurosis'. I think it would be better to view this as *bodily illness teaching the person how to be ill.* One's own sickness – and the responses of others to it, with which it is inextricably intermingled – becomes a model, or a rule, which one may later choose to follow or not follow. This is, then, one of the ways a person learns to follow rules that foster dependency by exhibiting signs of helplessness.

Such rules abound in religious, medical, and educational situations. Consequently, those exposed to them are subjected to pressures to adapt by assuming the required *postures of helplessness* (e.g. patients committed to state hospitals, candidates in psychoanalytic institutes, etc.). This leads to behaviour judged appropriate ('normal') within the system, but not necessarily outside it. Resistance to the rules may be tolerated to varying degrees in different systems, but in any event tends to bring the individual into conflict with the group. Hence, most persons seek to conform rather than to rebel. Another possibility for adaptation lies in becoming aware of the rules and of their limited, situational relevance. This makes it possible to get along in the system while it also allows one to maintain a large measure of inner freedom. To do this, however, requires a rather complex type of learning – that is learning about learning; and also resistance against being pressed into a role, even though role-acceptance might be richly rewarded.

What are the specific connections between these considerations and the problems posed by hysteria and mental illness?

If we regard psychiatry as the study of human behaviour, it is evident that it is intimately related to both ethics and politics. This relationship was already illustrated by means of several examples. Specifically with respect to hysteria, the connections between ethics and psychiatry may be highlighted by asking: *What kinds of human relationships and patterns of mastery does the so-called hysteric value?* Or, phrased somewhat differently: *What kind of (social) game does such a person want to play? And what sort of behaviour does he regard as playing the game well and winning?*

Before these questions can be answered, it will be necessary to inquire further into the nature of games. This, in turn, will require a logical classification of games, similar to that used for languages.

A Logical Hierarchy of Games

Until now, games have been treated as if they were all more or less of the same kind. This point of view will no longer suffice. Since games consist, among other things, of bits of communicative action, it is not surprising that a hierarchy of games analogous to a hierarchy of languages is easily constructed. Linguistic signs point to referents, such as physical objects, other words, or more complex systems of signs. Similarly, games consist of systems of rules which point to certain acts – the rules standing in the same relation to the acts as the words to their referents. Accordingly, games with rules that point to the simplest possible set of patterned acts will be called 'object games'. Games composed of rules which themselves point to other rules will be called 'metagames'. Typical examples of object games are patterns of instinctive behaviour. Their goals are physical survival, release of urinary, anal, or sexual tension, and so forth. Hence, playing object games is not limited to human beings. In the medical setting, the reflex immobilization of an injured extremity would be an example of a move in an object game.

It is obvious that *the learned and distinctively human elements of behaviour are entirely on the level of metagames.* Examples of first-level metagames are the rules determining *where to* urinate and *where not to*, *when to* eat and *when not to*, and so forth. Ordinary or conventional games – such as bridge, tennis, or chess – all comprise mixtures of complex metagames.

The Structure of Ordinary Games

Let us apply the concepts of game-hierarchy to the analysis of an ordinary game, say tennis. Like any game of skill and strategy, tennis is characterized by a set of basic rules which specify such things as the number of players, the layout of the court, the nature and use of rackets and balls, and so forth. Actually, although these rules are object-rules to tennis, they are metarules with respect to such logically anterior games as the proper laying out of courts, or the manufacturing of rackets. When we play tennis, however, we are not usually concerned with games lying on levels lower than the basic game of tennis itself. These infra-tennis games might, however, be important for those who want to play tennis but are prevented from doing so, say, by insufficient funds to purchase the necessary equipment.

Beginning at the level of the basic rules – assuming, that is, the presence of players, equipment, and so forth – it is evident that there is much more to an actual, true-to-life tennis game than could be subsumed under the basic rules. This is because there is more than one way to play tennis while still adhering to these rules which merely provide a minimal framework within which there is considerable latitude. For example, one player might aspire to winning at any cost; another to playing fairly. Each of these goals implies rules specifying, firstly, that in order to play tennis one must follow rules A, B, and C, and secondly, how one should conduct oneself while following these rules. The latter prescriptions constitute the rules of 'meta-tennis'. In everyday language, the term 'tennis' is used, of course, to denote *all* of the rules of this game. The fact that ordinary games may be played in more than one way – that is, that they contain games at different logical levels – leads to conflict whenever different types of players meet.

When two wildly competitive youngsters play tennis the game is so constituted that both players regard winning as their sole aim. Style, fair play, one's state of health, and everything else may become subordinated to this goal. In other words, the players play to win at any cost – adhering only to the appropriate basic rules of the game, such as placing shots within the prescribed area of the court, serving from the proper position, and so forth, and avoiding violating rules for which there are prescribed penalties.

A next higher level of tennis may be distinguished – a 'meta-tennis game', as it were – which, in addition to the basic rules, contains a new set of rules which refer to the basic rules. These might include prescriptions about style, the tempo of the game, courteous behaviour, etc. Playing according to higher level rules (metarules) implies, firstly, that the players will orient themselves to and follow a new set of rules, these being additional to, rather than substitutes for, the old set; and secondly, that the players will adopt as their own the new goals implicit in the new rules. In tennis, this might be to play fairly or perhaps elegantly, rather than to win at any cost. It is important to note now that the goals of the object game and of the metagame may come into conflict, although they need not necessarily do so. Adherence to the rules and aims (ethics) of the higher level game usually implies that its rules and goals take precedence over those of the basic game. In other words, for a properly socialized Englishman, it is better – that is, more rewarding in relation to both the spectators and his own self-image – to be a 'fair loser' than an 'ugly winner'. But if this is true, then our everyday use of the words 'loser' and 'winner' *no longer do justice to what we want to say*. For when we speak of James as a 'fair loser', especially if he is contrasted with an opponent considered an 'ugly winner', what we mean is that James lost the basic game but has won the metagame. But we cannot say anything like this in ordinary language – except by circumlocution – for example, by saying that 'James played a good game but lost.'

Everyday Life as a Mixture of Metagames

Everyday life is full of situations similar to the example sketched above. *Men are constantly engaged in behaviour involving complicated mixtures of various logical levels of games.* Unless the precise games which men play are clarified – and also, whether they play them well, badly, or indifferently – there is little chance of understanding what 'is actually going on' or of altering it.

Let us ask: What rules do men actually follow in their daily lives? The metaphorical net which this question throws out is so wide that it catches too much. Let us, therefore, narrow it down to the case of a 'simple man'. We seek to understand only the basic rules of living, and only one version of them: for example, the biblical rules of life. The Ten Commandments may then be likened to the directions one receives when purchasing a new appliance. The buyer is told that he must follow certain rules if he wants to derive the benefits the machine has to offer. If he fails to follow the directions, he will have to suffer the consequences. In the case of breakdowns, for example, the manufacturer's warranty is honoured only if the machine has not been misused. Here is a fitting analogy for legitimate illness (manufacturing defect), as contrasted to sin or other types of unallowed illness (misuse of the machine). The Ten Commandments – and biblical teachings generally – are the rules man must follow if he expects to obtain the benefits which the manufacturer of the game of life (God) offers the purchaser (man).

However, in the case of real-life games, the situation is more complicated. It often happens that the game rules instruct the player that in order to 'win' he must 'lose'. In this connection, let us recall some of the biblical rules discussed in Chapter 9; for example, the following two prescriptions for 'good living': (1) 'Blessed *are* the meek: for they shall inherit the earth' (Matthew 5:5); (2) 'Blessed *are* they which are persecuted for righteousness' sake: for theirs is the kingdom of heaven' (Matthew 5:10).

I submit that a basic assumption underlies these rules – namely, that it *happens* that some people are meek and that others are persecuted. Being meek and persecuted are tacitly assumed to be occurrences not deliberately sought. But are they not? And might they not be?

In the days of early Christianity, much as today, aggressive men often tended to get the better of their less aggressive neighbours. Apparently, ethical rules came into being in an effort to provide for the sort of thing which the British call fair play. This, however, complicated matters considerably, for games of increasingly higher orders were thus created.

Looking, then, at problems in living from this point of view, it seems apparent that much of what goes by the names of 'growing up', 'becoming sophisticated', 'getting treated by psychoanalysis' (and by other methods as well) are processes having one significant feature in common: *the person learns that the rules of the game – and the very game itself – by which he has been playing are not necessarily the same as those used by others around him.* He thus learns that others may not be interested in playing the game which he has been so avidly pursuing. Or, if they do have some interest in the game, they prefer some modifications of the rules. Thus, unless a person finds others to play his own game, according to his own rules – or wishes and is able to coerce others to accept life on his terms[2] – he has a choice among three basic alternatives.

One is to submit to the other person's coercive rules and accept the masochistic-submissive posture offered.

The second is increasingly to renounce socially shared activities and to withdraw into certain relatively idiosyncratic games. Such activities may be labelled scientific, artistic, religious, neurotic, or psychotic, depending on various, generally poorly defined criteria. The nature of these criteria need not concern us here, but we should note that the issue of *social utility* plays a significant role in it. In turn, this raises further questions: for whom (i.e. for what persons), and at what time (in history), is a particular game useful?

The third is to become aware of one's own games, as well as those of others, and to try to make compromises among them.

[2] This point of view makes the significant connections between mental illness and social class very clear, especially as it relates to the issue of *power*. In other words, persons who wield vast power have the opportunity, by and large, to coerce others to play their own games. And as long as they can do this, they *cannot* become 'mentally ill' in a social sense (Szasz, 1958f, 1960c).

This is an arduous undertaking which often can be, at best, only partly successful. Its main reward lies in guaranteeing the integrity and dignity of one's own self and of all others with whom one interacts. Yet its hardships are such that it need not surprise us if many prefer easier means leading to what must appear, to them, as more important ends.

What are we to believe when a person insists that he is playing game A, but observation reveals that he is following the rules of game B? We might conclude, firstly, that the player really believes that he is playing game A, even though he is not, perhaps because he has failed properly to distinguish between game A and game B; or, secondly, that he is deliberately cheating, that is, he knows the rules of game A perfectly well but has chosen to violate them in the hope of enhancing his chances to win. It is important to keep in mind that the player who cheats has not given up playing game A, for he continues to be committed to its end-goal, namely, winning. He has simply modified the rules, but has kept this rule-changing private – or secret! *This non-codification of the new rules is the most distinguishing characteristic of cheating.* These observations underscore the significance of publicity in regard to game rules.

The phenomena I shall discuss in this chapter could be conceptualized several ways – as cheating, sickness, stupidity, or sin. By analysing them in terms of a game model of behaviour, it will be possible to bring order and harmony to such apparently diverse and unrelated phenomena as lying, cheating, making a mistake, malingering, the Ganser syndrome, and imposturing.

The Concept of Impersonation

Impersonation refers to a large class of events characterized by the assumption of another person's character or social role. It is a ubiquitous occurrence and does not constitute a specifically psychiatric problem. Indeed, there are, in everyday language, numerous words to designate different kinds of impersonations. As nouns, denoting the impersonator, we have the charlatan, the confidence-man, the counterfeiter, the forger, the impostor, the quack, the spy, the traitor, and so forth. Two types of impersonators, the malingerer and the hysteric, have been of special interest to psychiatrists.

A definition of impersonation is now in order. According to Webster, to impersonate is 'to assume or act the person or character of ...'. This definition provokes some interesting difficulties: if role-taking behaviour is universal, how do we distinguish role-taking (in Mead's sense) from impersonation (in common-sense usage)? I would offer the following answer: *role-taking refers to consistent or honest role-playing, within the limits of a specific game, whereas impersonation refers to the pretended assumption of a role, manifested by inconsistent or dishonest role-playing.* For example, taking the role of 'vendor' and approaching another person as a prospective customer implies that the seller either owns the goods offered for sale, or is authorized to act in the owner's name. When a person sells something he does not own, he impersonates the role of an honest vendor and is called a 'swindler'.

Since role-taking is a permanent and universal characteristic of human behaviour, it is evident that practically any action can be *interpreted* as a type of impersonation. For example, the so-called Don Juan may be said to impersonate a man of acrobatic virility; the transvestite, the social role and sexual functions of a member of the opposite sex; and so forth.

Impersonation in Childhood

A great deal of childhood is spent in impersonating others. Children play at being fireman, doctor, nurse, mother, father. Inasmuch as the child's identity is defined in predominantly negative terms – that is, in terms of what he *cannot do*, because he is not allowed to do it or is incapable of doing it – it is not surprising that he should seek role-fulfilment through impersonation. A child's real identity or social role is, of course, to be a child. But in an achievement-oriented culture, as opposed to a tradition- and kinship-oriented one, being a child tends to mean mostly that one is unable or unfit to act in certain ways. Thus, childhood itself may be viewed as a form of disability.[1]

Let us reconsider the impersonations engaged in by children, say, between the ages of four and ten. In these activities the observers (i.e. the grown-ups) have no difficulty recognizing the pretended, or impersonated, character of the role. This is because a child playing doctor or nurse presents a cognitive task of such utter simplicity that any adult who is not an imbecile could not help but master it. It is partly the child's size of course, which helps so decisively to give him an identity: he is small. Contrast this, for example, with the case of a psychologist practising psychotherapy. For many people, such a person is indistinguishable from a doctor or psychiatrist. To distinguish between medical and non-medical psychotherapists, one must have certain specific kinds of information. In this case, one cannot rely on the person's size, skin colour, or other equally easily ascertainable characteristics for help in differentiating between two similar types of activities.

Impersonation, then, is a ubiquitous feature of childhood. The notions of imitation, identification, and learning refer either to the same thing as impersonation or to what may be regarded as component parts of it. And the problem of successful impersonation, for the reasons just noted, does not arise until after puberty and the attainment of physiological maturity.

Psychiatric and psychoanalytic authors have systematically failed to distinguish between a general class of events, called impersonations, and certain members of this class, for example imposturing. Helene Deutsch (1942, 1955), in particular, has confused or equated the impostor and the impersonator. Some of her observations apply to imposturing, others to impersonating. The following passage (H. Deutsch, 1955) is illustrative:

The world is crowded with 'as-if' personalities, and even more so with impostors and pretenders. Ever since I became interested in the impostor, he pursues me everywhere. I find him among my friends and acquaintances, as well as in myself. Little Nancy, a fine $3\frac{1}{2}$-year-old daughter of one of my friends, goes around with an air of dignity,

[1] Similar considerations hold for the aged. As old persons become unemployed and unproductive, and particularly if they are economically and physically disabled, their main role becomes being old.

holding her hands together tightly. Asked about this attitude she explains: 'I am Nancy's guardian angel, and I'm taking care of little Nancy.' Her father asked her about the angel's name; 'Nancy' was the proud answer of this little impostor. (p. 503)

Deutsch correctly observed that the world is full of people who act 'as if' they were someone else. Alfred Adler (1914) emphasized this phenomenon much earlier and called it the 'life-lie'. In this connection, we might also recall Vaihinger's work, *The Philosophy of 'As If'* (1911), which influenced both Freud's and Adler's theories.

The point to be emphasized is that not all impersonators are impostors, but that all impostors are impersonators. In illustrating impersonation, 'which she erroneously called imposturing, Deutsch cited examples on the behaviour of children. But, as we saw, children *must* impersonate others because they are *nobodies*. In her conclusion, Deutsch (1955) suggested that the essence of imposturing lay in 'pretending that we actually are what we would like to be' (p. 504). But this is merely a restatement of the common human desire to appear better than one actually is. It is not a correct formulation of imposturing, which implies deceitful role-taking for personal gain. Impersonation is a morally more neutral name for a class that contains both morally objectionable and unobjectionable types of role-pretensions.

The desire to be better or more important than one is is likely to be strongest, of course, among children, or among persons who are, or consider themselves to be, in inferior, oppressed, or frustrating circumstances.[2] These are the same persons who are most likely to resort to various methods of impersonation. Conversely, those who have been successful in realizing their aspirations – who, in other words, are relatively well satisfied with their actual role achievements and definitions – will be unlikely to pretend to be anyone but themselves. They are satisfied with who they are and can afford the luxury of telling the truth about themselves.

[2] I do not wish to imply that children are invariably oppressed or that their lack of a firm inner identity is due to 'oppression'. Indeed, the role of being oppressed can itself be the core of one's identity. The lack of firm personal identity in childhood is a reflection mainly of the child's insufficient social and psychological development.

Varieties of Impersonation

Lying

The simplest and best understood example of impersonation is lying. This term is used usually in relation to verbal or written communication; and only when it is assumed that the communicants have pledged themselves to truthfulness. Thus, the term 'lying' can be used meaningfully only when the rules of the game call for truthfulness. This condition obtains in many human relationships, especially in those that are emotionally close, such as marriage and friendship. Perjury is a special kind of lying, committed in a court of law by a person giving testimony. Here the rules of the game are explicitly formulated; lying is punishable by legally enforced sanctions.

Cheating

Cheating means rule-deviance in situations explicitly codified as games, usually serving the purpose of unfairly increasing the player's chances of winning. In addition to this strict usage, 'cheating' is also used more loosely to describe deceit or imposture of various kinds. A person may be 'cheated' in a business venture, or a husband by his wife. In all these situations where we speak of cheating, the rules of the game are known to all concerned.

The maxim, 'Ignorance of the law is no excuse', is pertinent in this connection. This ground rule of Anglo-American law asserts that *it is the responsibility of every adult to know what kind of games the state requires him to play*. In this view, being ignorant of the law is tantamount to not being a fully socialized person.

When knowledge of the rules of the game might be lacking, or when its status is uncertain – for example, in psychiatry and politics – we usually do not speak of cheating, but instead create concepts such as 'hysteria' or 'patriotism'. Since a great deal of human behaviour may be regarded as if it were a kind of game, the scope of the word 'cheating' may be greatly expanded. Conceptualizing some of our traditional psychiatric problems in this way, it becomes apparent that many of these have little in common with bodily illnesses, but much with cheating.

Malingering

Cheating is impersonating the correctly behaving player. Malingering is impersonating the correctly sick person. What constitutes correct sickness depends, of course, on the rules of the particular *illness* game, a subject discussed earlier (e.g. Chapter 1). It is the element of rule awareness that must be emphasized here. A person who knew nothing about the rules of the sickness game could not malinger. This is a truism. It is like asserting that someone who did not know that Picasso's canvases were valuable could not, and hence would not, try to sell a forged Picasso for a large sum of money. This still leaves us with the problem of self-deception and error.

For instance, a person might truly believe that he was bodily ill when in fact he was not, and might then represent himself as sick. Such an individual resembles a person who has unknowingly purchased a good imitation of a Picasso, believing it to be an original, and who subsequently represents it and tries to sell it as a Picasso. Obviously there is a difference between this man and the one who actually paints the imitation and then misrepresents it. Malingering has, as I noted, been usually conceptualized as deliberate cheating, and hysteria as unwitting or unintentional cheating. My aim here is to describe both as impersonation. Whether the impersonation is conscious and deliberate or otherwise may be ascertained by communicating with the person, and by making inferences from his behaviour.

Hysteria, Hypochondriasis, and Bodily Delusions

Special instances of impersonation are encountered in hysteria, hypochondriasis, and severe cases of bodily delusions (e.g. in schizophrenia). In hysteria, the patient impersonates the role of a sick person, in part by identifying with and displaying his symptoms. Allegedly, however, he does not know that he is doing so. When it is said that the hysteric cannot afford to be aware of what he is doing – for if he were, he could no longer do it – what is asserted in effect is that he cannot afford to tell himself the truth. By the same token, he also cannot afford to know that he is lying. He must lie both to himself and to others.

This view underscores the importance of the connections between opression, helplessness, and the use of hysterical and other types of indirect communications. To be able to speak the truth is a luxury which few people can afford. This we often forget. *To be able to be truthful one must be more or less grown up and personally secure, and one must live in a social situation which encourages, or at least permits, truthfulness.* We often assume – and this is an error – that truthful communications are everywhere encouraged and rewarded and that lying and cheating are everywhere discouraged and penalized. I tried to identify the conditions that favour the mendacity and cheating which we call hysteria.

Hypochondriasis and schizophrenic bodily delusions are additional examples of consciously unrecognized impersonations of bodily illness. Thus, a person's claim that he is dying, or that he is dead, is best regarded as an impersonation of the dead role. Of course, the less public support there is for an impersonation, the more unreflective the impersonator must be to maintain it. Indeed, the label of psychosis is often used to identify individuals who stubbornly cling to, and loudly proclaim, publicly unsupported role-definitions.

The Ganser Syndrome

This phenomenon, to be examined more fully presently, consists of the strategic impersonation of the 'crazy role' by a prisoner. There is a great deal of psychiatric controversy regarding the nature of this alleged illness, and whether it is akin to malingering, hysteria, or psychosis (Arieti and Meth, 1959). I suggest that this phenomenon be cast in the framework of the *prison-plus-sickness game* and that it be considered a special, strikingly transparent, form of impersonation or cheating.

The Confidence Man

The confidence man impersonates a role that usually inspires trust. In the longer run, however, whoever trusts him will be deceived. The impersonation is for selfish gain and is not openly acknowledged to the victim, although it may be to the self and to others (Mann, 1954; Maurer, 1950). 'Confidence games' are so played that the gains to the impersonator, and the losses to those he swindles, are evident, at least in retrospect.

Theatrical Impersonation

Finally, I want to say a few words about theatrical impersonation. Here, impersonation occurs in a special social setting which explicitly identifies role-taking as impersonation. For example, if an actor plays the role of Abraham Lincoln, the audience is informed, by means of appropriate messages, that the man who looks and talks like Lincoln is only taking his role for the purposes of the play. This is a very special type of impersonation in that *all* of the participants in the game are explicitly aware that it *is* impersonation. Nevertheless, it has much in common with the other types discussed.

The foregoing is not intended as a complete list of all known types of impersonations. It is impossible to prepare such a list, for there are as many impersonations as there are roles. We touch here also on the much discussed subject of *identity*, and its underlying psychological mechanism, *identification*. In the existential analytic conceptions of *authentic* and *inauthentic existences* we encounter a similar concern – that is, with whether a state of being is genuine or impersonated. Authentic existence is life-role consciously and responsibly assumed, while in-authentic existence is role foisted on the person and only passively accepted by him. It is clear, therefore, that the notions of existence, role, and game are closely related. Current psycho-analytic studies concerned with identity, existential-analytic interest in authentic life patterns, and semiotical and game-analytic inquiry into behaviour all point to certain common problems and similar attempts to solve them.

The Ganser Syndrome

The Ganser syndrome, which is usually considered to be a variant of either malingering or hysteria, provides an excellent

229

illustration of the need to abandon the medical-pathological frame of reference in psychiatry and to substitute a communicational and game-playing model for it.

In 1898 a German psychiatrist, S. Ganser, described what he called a 'specific hysterical twilight state', the chief symptom of which he identified as *Vorbeireden*. This was subsequently named *paralogia*, or the syndrome of approximate answers. According to Noyes (1956) this alleged syndrome is characterized by the following features:

An interesting type of *mental disorder* sometimes occurring in the case of prisoners under detention awaiting trial was described by Ganser. It develops only after commission of a crime and, therefore, tells nothing about the patient's mental state when he committed the offence. In this *syndrome*, the *patient*, being under charges from which he would be exonerated were he *irresponsible*, begins, *without being aware of the fact*, to appear *irresponsible*. He appears stupid and unable to comprehend questions or instructions accurately. His replies are vaguely relevant to the query but absurd in content. He performs various uncomplicated, familiar tasks in an absurd manner, or gives approximate replies to simple questions. The patient, for example, may attempt to write with the blunt end of his pencil, or will give 11 as the product of 4×3. *The purpose of the patient's behaviour is so obviously to appear irresponsible that the inexperienced observer frequently believes that he is malingering. The dynamics is probably that of a dissociative process.* ([Italics added] pp. 505–6)

It should be noted that, in this account, the person exhibiting this sort of conduct is labelled a 'patient', and his behaviour a 'mental disorder'. But how has it been shown that he is 'sick'?

Here is another interpretation – this one by Wertham (1949) – of the Ganser syndrome:

A Ganser reaction is a hysterical pseudo-stupidity which occurs almost exclusively in jails and in old-fashioned German textbooks. It is now *known* to be almost always due more to *conscious malingering* than to unconscious stupefaction. ([Italics added] p. 191)

If the Ganser 'patient' impersonates what he thinks is the behaviour of the mentally sick – to plead irresponsibility and avoid punishment – how does his behaviour differ from that of a person who cheats on his income tax return? As the former feigns stupidity, so the latter feigns poverty. It seems to me logically completely unjustified to regard this type of behaviour as a form of illness (Weiner and Braiman, 1955).

Let us now examine the sort of impersonation encountered here and its similarities to other types of role-taking. It is astonishing how well persons exhibiting the typical features of the Ganser syndrome – and so-called malingerers and hysterics, too – have succeeded in convincing both themselves and those around them that they are, in fact, *sick* (meaning by this, disabled, not responsible, perhaps even bodily ill). Their success in this regard is proved by the fact that according to both professional and popular opinion these forms of human conduct are increasingly viewed and accepted as instances of *genuine* illness. This, of course, is exactly the impression which those who act thus wish to create. But in accepting this imagery, both they and we are misled and confused.

An analogy from the world of the theatre might help to clarify this situation. The terms 'type-casting' and 'becoming typed' describe how an actor who frequently appears in the same type of role soon creates the impression in the public that he 'really' is like the person or character type he has been portraying. One thinks, in this connection, of the actors who have been 'typed' as bad men or of the actresses who have been publicly defined as sex-bombs. For Americans, the Frankenstein monster is Boris Karloff, Abraham Lincoln is Raymond Massey, and F.D.R. is Ralph Bellamy. The actors' assumed identities may prove convincing not only to their audiences but to themselves as well. They may then begin to act offstage as if they were on it.

The crux of this analogy between type-casting and the impersonation of the sick role in hysteria and allied disorders is that, psychiatric arguments to the contrary, it does make a difference whether a role is impersonated or whether it is genuine. This statement requires explanation along two lines. Firstly, it might be argued that if a person does not know that he is playing a false role, then his role must be regarded as genuine. It will be shown, however, that there are other bases than self-awareness for judging this matter. Secondly, it must be kept in mind that the actor and the audience (i.e. patient and physician, or relatives) occupy two different, albeit complementary, sectors of a larger field. Impersonation and genuine role are defined sometimes by the actor, sometimes by the audience, and often by an agreement of both.

Roles : Assumed, Impersonated, and Genuine

The Assumed Role Becomes Believable and is Accepted

When the so-called malingerer or hysteric or Ganser syndrome patient becomes codified as 'sick' – even if mentally sick – he has succeeded in making his assumed role believable and accepted. This phenomenon, encountered in many human relationships, should be regarded in the same way as is the 'typing' of an actor. There is nothing especially unusual about this. We assume that our knowledge and image of the world around us is built up on the basis of our actual experiences. As the proverb has it, 'seeing is believing'. But we also know that sense impressions cannot always be taken at face value. They require critical scrutiny, checking, validation, comparison with the experiences of others, and so forth. This, then, raises the issue of complementary channels of information: a person can be critical of his impressions or information only if he has more than one way to find out about something. For example, by listening *only* it may be impossible to distinguish between the actual singing of a person and a recording of his voice. Listening *and* looking easily resolves the problem.

In the case of the so-called Ganser syndrome, by defining this type of behaviour as a form of mental illness psychiatrists confirm and verify the sufferer's definition of himself as sick. It is as if a theatre audience accepted Raymond Massey as Abraham Lincoln and began to treat him as president of the United States. Obviously, this sort of response feeds back to the actor (patient), for whom it means, in effect, that he can no longer rely on his audience for another, more realistic definition of his identity. This is a contingency with which few persons reckon when they launch themselves on a career of impersonating the sick role.

As a rule, persons assuming impersonated roles count on some resistance against their role-taking. Malingerers, for instance, expect to be opposed by physicians; swindlers by those whom they have swindled and by the legal machinery of society; and so forth. In general, the audience's resistance to the actor's taking an impersonated role is strongest at the beginning of a 'performance'. After an initial phase, the impersonated role is either repudiated or accepted. Once it is accepted, it is scrutinized much less than it was formerly. We are all familiar with this phenomenon. Once a schoolboy is regarded as a good student, the teachers will scrutinize his performance much less strictly than the bad student's. Similarly, actors, athletes, financiers, and others of *proved ability* are much more immune to criticism than those not so accepted.

In taking a role, then, the main task is to put on a good performance. If the performance pertains to an instrumentally defined task – that is, to a genuine role – its mastery means successful role-playing, and failure means unsuccessful role-playing. If, however, the performance involves impersonation, the possibilities for failure are doubled: the person may fail, firstly, by putting on an inadequate performance, thus having his role-pretension repudiated; and, secondly, by putting on a performance that is only too convincing, thus succeeding in making his impersonated role accepted.

We saw how this happens to some actors. In general, this hazard threatens only the successful performer, or one who has been well accepted in a particular role. Similarly, being called a malingerer and having one's sick-role aspirations repudiated is a danger facing only the beginner in this game. The person who impersonates the sick role and whose impersonation is successful resembles the actor who has been so convincing in his theatrical performances that his role is mistaken for his real identity. I submit that this is the status of most persons we call 'mentally ill'. By and large, such persons impersonate[3] the roles of helplessness, hopelessness, weakness, and often of bodily illness – when, in fact, their actual roles pertain to frustrations, unhappinesses, and perplexities due to interpersonal, social, and ethical conflicts.

[3] I do not wish to imply that this impersonation is always a consciously planned strategy, arrived at by deliberate choice among several alternatives – although, sometimes, it clearly is.

I have tried to point out the dangers which threaten certain impersonators (e.g. the mentally ill), as well as those who accept their impersonation (e.g. psychiatrists, the general public, etc.) – the main danger being the creation of a culturally shared *folie*, or myth. I believe that 'mental illness' is such a myth.

From Repudiation of 'Mental Illness' as Illness to its Acceptance

Contemporary psychiatry reflects the dangers characteristic of a late stage in the mental illness game. In its earlier stages – that is, in the days of Charcot, Breuer, and Freud – when most psychiatrists were neurologists and neuropathologists, psychiatrists were violently opposed to impersonations of the sick role. They wanted to see only 'really' sick – that is, neurologically sick – patients. They believed, therefore, that all mental patients were fakers and frauds.

Now psychiatrists have swung to the opposite extreme. They refuse to distinguish impersonated from genuine roles – cheating from playing honestly. In so conducting themselves, they act like the art expert mentioned earlier, who decides that a good imitation of a masterpiece is also an 'original masterpiece'.

Conceptualizing psychiatric illness on the model of medical illness, psychiatrists leave themselves no choice but to define psychiatric treatment as something that can be 'given' only to persons who 'have' a psychiatric illness! This leads not only to further unmanageable complications in conceptualizing the true nature of so-called psychiatric diseases and treatments, but also to an absurd dilemma with regard to persons who impersonate the role of the mentally sick patient.

Once a role is socially accepted, it must, in principle at least, be possible to imitate or impersonate it. The question then is: How shall the person who impersonates the role of mental patient be regarded – as malingering insanity or as insane? Psychiatrists wanted to claim such persons as patients so that they could 'treat' them. They could do so only if those who pretended to be mentally sick were also conceptualized and defined as 'sick'; hence, they were.

Thus, without perhaps anyone fully realizing just what was happening, the boundaries between the psychiatric game and the real life game became increasingly blurred. The lonely, romantic movie fan, enchanted with his idolized actress on the screen, may gradually come to feel that she is actually becoming a close, lifelike, and intimate figure. What is needed for this is a convincing performance and a receptive audience. But just as men need a Marilyn Monroe, or women a Clark Gable, so *physicians need sick people*! I submit, therefore, that anyone who acts sick – impersonating this role – and does so vis-à-vis persons who are therapeutically inclined, runs the risk of being accepted in his impersonated role. And in being so accepted he endangers himself in certain, often unexpected, ways. Although ostensibly he is requesting and receiving help, what is called 'help' might be forthcoming only if he accepts the sick role and all that it may imply for his therapist.

The principal alternative to this dilemma lies, as I suggested before, *in abolishing the categories of ill and healthy behaviour*, and the prerequisite of mental sickness for so-called psychotherapy. This implies candid recognition that we 'treat' people by psychoanalysis or psychotherapy not because they are 'sick' but, firstly, because they desire this type of assistance; secondly, because they have problems in living for which they seek mastery through understanding of the kinds of games which they, and those around them, have been in the habit of playing; and, thirdly, because as psychotherapists we want and are able to participate in their 'education', this being our professional role.

Some Differences between Impersonated and Genuine Roles

The concept of an impersonated role has meaning only in contrast with a genuine role. The method for differentiating impersonated or false roles from genuine or real ones is the familiar process of *verification*. This may be a social process, consisting of the comparison of opinions from various observers (Goffman, 1959, pp. 60–65). Or it may be a scientifically more distinctive operation, consisting of testing assertions or hypotheses against observations or experiments. In its simplest forms, verification involves no more than the use of complementary channels of information – for example, sight and hearing, checking the patient's statements against certain official documents, etc. Let us consider the case of a person who claims to be Jesus. If you ask such a person for evidence to support his claim, he may say that he suffers and soon expects to die, or that his mother is the Virgin Mary. Of course, we will not believe him.

This, however, is a crude and trivial example. It fails to confront us with the more subtle and difficult problems in validating roles, such as occur characteristically with persons who complain of pain. Here the question becomes: Does the patient 'really' have pain – that is, *is he a genuine occupant of the sick role*? Or is his pain 'hysterical' – that is, due, for example, to identification with someone who had a similar complaint – and hence *does he impersonate the sick role*? In this sort of case we cannot rely on asking other people whether they think that the patient is 'sick' or 'malingers'. The criterion for differentiating between the two roles must be scientific rather than social. In other words, it will be necessary to perform certain 'operations' or 'tests' to secure more information on which to base further inferences. In the case of differentiating bodily from mental illness, the principal method for gathering further information is the physical, laboratory, and psychological examination of the patient.

Viewing impersonation and genuine role-playing in terms of games, they could be said to represent two fundamentally different games. In genuine role-playing, the actor commits himself to the game with the goal of playing as well as he can: for example, the surgeon tries to cure the sick person by the proper removal of the diseased organ. In impersonated role-playing the actor commits himself to imitating the well-playing person: for example, the man who impersonates a physician tries to convince people that he is one so that he can enjoy the economic and social rewards of the physician's role.

In impersonation, then, the goal is to look like the imitated person or role-performance; that is, to effect an outward, or 'superficial', similarity between self and other. This may be achieved by dress, manner of speech, symptom, making certain claims, and so forth. Why some persons seek role-imitation rather than competence and task-mastery need not concern us here.

The desire for unnecessary surgical operations – 'unnecessary', that is, from the point of view of pathophysiology – is often a part of the strategy of impersonation. In this situation, the impersonator plays the illness game and tries to validate his claim to the sick role. The surgeon who consents to operate on such persons performs a useful function for them, albeit his usefulness cannot be justified on surgical grounds. His intervention *legitimizes the 'patient's' claim to the sick role*. The surgical scar is official proof of illness: it is the diploma that proves the genuineness of patienthood.

In genuine role-playing, on the other hand, the individual's purpose, usually consciously entertained, is to acquire certain skills or knowledge. The desire for a certain kind of similarity to another person – say, to a surgeon or scientist – may be operative here also. But the goals as well as the rules of this game require that the similarity be substantive rather than superficial. The goal is learning, and hence an alteration of the 'inner personality' rather than a mere 'outer change' such as occurs in impersonation.

The distinction between genuine and impersonated roles may be described in still another way, by making use of the concepts of instrumental and institutional groups and the criteria for membership in them. *Instrumental groups* are based on shared skills. Membership in them, say in a Davis Cup team, implies that the person possesses a special skill. We consider this role genuine because such a person really knows how to play tennis. *Institutional groups*, on the other hand, are based on kinship, status, and other non-functional criteria. Membership in a family, say in a royal family, is an example. When the king dies, the crown prince becomes the new king. This transformation from non-king to king requires no new knowledge or skills; it requires only being the son of a dead king.

Impersonation may be summed up in one sentence, as a strategy of behaviour based on the model of hereditary monarchies. Implicit in this strategy is a deepseated belief that instrumental skills are unimportant. All that is needed to succeed in the game of life is to 'play a role' and gain social approval for it. Parents often hold up this model for their children to follow.

When they do follow it, they soon end up with an 'empty' life. When the child or young adult then tries to fill the void, his efforts to do so are often labelled some form of 'mental illness'. However, being 'mentally ill' or 'psychotic' – or killing someone else or himself – may be the only games left for such a person to play.

13 Hysteria as a Game

By slightly modifying Piaget's (1932, 1951) scheme of the development of the capacity to follow and to be aware of rules, I propose to distinguish *three stages, or types, of mastery of interpersonal processes*: coercion, self-help, and co-operation. This series constitutes a developmental sequence. Coercion is the simplest rule to follow, the easiest game to play; self-help is the next most difficult; and co-operation is the most demanding of them all.

Coercion, Self-Help and Co-operation in Hysteria

The hysteric plays a game in which there is an unequal mixture of coercive, self-helping, and co-operative strategies. While coercive manoeuvres predominate, elements of self-help and co-operation are not completely lacking. A distinct achievement of this type of behaviour is a synthesis of sorts among three separate and to some extent conflicting games, values, and styles of life. In this lies its strength as well as its weakness.

Because of this inner contradiction in the hysteric's life-game, he fails to play well at any one of three games. To begin with, the hysteric places a high value on *coercive strategies*. True, he may not be aware that he has made a choice between coercion and other strategies. His wish to coerce others may be 'unconscious'. Usually, however, it is not so much unconscious as it is inexplicit. In psychotherapy, it is generally easily recognized by the therapist and readily acknowledged by the patient. The point to be emphasized here is that although the hysteric espouses the value of coercion and domination he cannot play this game in a skilful and uninhibited manner. To do so requires two qualities he lacks: a relatively indiscriminating identification with the aggressor, and a large measure of insensitivity to the needs and feelings of others. The hysteric has too much compassion to play the game of domination openly and successfully. *He can coerce and dominate with suffering, but not with 'selfish' will.*

To play the game of self-help well requires *committing* one's self to it. This often leads to isolation from others: human relationships are not strongly cultivated. Religious, artistic, or other work investments displace interest in personal relationships. Playing well at this game is highly rewarded in our culture. Preoccupation with one's body or with suffering and helplessness interferes, of course, with one's ability to concentrate on the practical tasks that must be mastered to play such games well. Moreover, the tactic of dominating others by displaying helplessness cannot be maintained unaltered in the face of a high degree of demonstrable competence in important areas of life. The aim of coercing others by exhibiting helplessness may still be retained but the tactics by which this goal is pursued must be modified. The proverbial absent-minded professor is a case in point. Here is a composite of the famous scientist, highly skilled in his complex work performance, who is at the same time as helpless as a child when it comes to feeding himself, putting on his boots, or paying his income tax. Exhibitions of helplessness in these areas invite help in exactly the same manner in which bodily complaints invite medical attention.

Finally, the game of co-operation, implies and requires a value which the person exhibiting hysterical symptoms may not share at all. I believe that in hysteria, we are confronted with a genuine *clash of values – namely, between equality and co-operativeness on the one hand, and inequality and domination–submission on the other.* This conflict of values actually takes place in two distinct spheres: in the intrapersonal system of the patient and in the interpersonal system of therapy.

In psychiatry, the problem of hysteria is not formulated in this way. Psychiatrists prefer to operate with the tacit assumption that whatever their values are they are the same values that their patients hold and their colleagues share! Of course, this cannot always be the case. If, however, value conflicts of this sort are as important in psychiatry as I am suggesting why are they not made explicit? The answer is simple: because doing so *threatens the cohesion of the group* – that is, the prestige and the power of the psychiatric profession.

Hysteria as a Mixture of Conflicting Values and Disparate Games

The idea that hysterical symptoms (as well as other neurotic symptoms) are compromises is a cornerstone of psychoanalytic theory. Early in his work, Freud thought in terms of compromise formations between instinctual drives and social defences, or between selfish needs and the requirements of communal living. Later, he asserted that neuroses were due to conflicts and compromises between id and ego, or id and superego. I now want to describe hysteria as still another compromise, this time among three different types of games.

Typical of the *coercive game* we call 'hysteria' is the powerful promotive impact of iconic body signs on those to whom they are directed. The patient's relatives, for example, tend to be deeply impressed by such communications, often much more deeply than they would be by similar statements framed in ordinary language. The display of sickness or suffering is thus useful for coercing others. This feature of hysteria, more than any other, accounts for its immediate and immense practical value to the patient.

The game of *self-help* is also present in most cases of hysteria. Classically, hysterical patients were said to exhibit an attitude of indifference towards their suffering. This manifest indifference signifies, firstly, a denial that the patient has in fact made a coercive communication and, secondly, an affirmation that the patient aspires to a measure of self-sufficiency. Hysterics are thus not wholly coercive in their relationship to others but are, to some extent, self-reliant and self-sufficient. However, they can attend to their self-helping strategies only half-heartedly, being ready to coerce by means of symptoms should other methods of mastery fail. Learning new tactics of self-help or co-operation is difficult for them and is often not encouraged in the social setting in which they live.

Hysterics play the *co-operative game* very imperfectly. This is to be expected, as this game requires and presupposes a feeling of relative equality among the players. Persons employing hysterical methods of communication feel – and often are – inferior and oppressed. In turn they aspire to feeling superior to others and to oppressing them. But they also seek equality of sorts and some measure of co-operation as potential remedies for their oppressed status.

Hysteria is thus mainly a coercive game, with small elements of self-help and still smaller elements of co-operation blended in. This view implies that the hysteric is unclear about his values and their connection with his behaviour.

We might again note here that several of the patients reported in the early psychoanalytic literature were young women who became 'ill' with hysteria while caring for a sick, usually older, relative. This was true in the case of Breuer's (Breuer and Freud, 1893–5) famous patient, Anna O.:

In July 1880, the patient's father, of whom she was passionately fond, fell ill of a peripleuritic abscess which failed to clear up and to which he succumbed in April 1881. During the first months of the illness Anna devoted her whole energy to nursing her father, and no one was much surprised when by degrees her own health greatly deteriorated. No one, perhaps not even the patient herself, knew what was happening to her; but eventually the state of weakness, anaemia and distaste for food became so bad that *to her great sorrow she was no longer allowed to continue nursing the patient.* ([Italics added] pp. 22–3)

Anna O. thus started to play the hysterical game from a position of distasteful submission: she functioned as an oppressed, unpaid, sick-nurse, *who was coerced to be helpful by the very helplessness of a (bodily) sick patient.* The women in Anna O.'s position were – as are their counterparts today, who feel similarly entrapped by their small children – insufficiently aware of what they valued in life and of how their own ideas of what they valued affected their conduct. For example, young middle-class women in Freud's day considered it their duty to take care of their sick fathers. Hiring a professional servant or nurse for this job would have created a moral conflict for them, because it would have symbolized to them as well as to others that they did not love ('care for') their fathers. Similarly, many contemporary American women find themselves enslaved by their young children. Today, married women are generally expected to take care of their own children; they are not supposed to delegate this task to others. The 'old folks' can be placed in a home; it is all right to delegate their care to hired help. This is a complete reversal of the social situation which prevailed in upper- and middle-class European circles until the First World War and even after it. Then, children were often cared for by hired help, while parents were taken care of by their children, now fully grown.

In both situations, the *obligatory* nature of the care required generates a feeling of helplessness in the person from whom help is sought. If a person cannot, in good conscience, refuse to provide help – and cannot even stipulate the terms on which he will supply it – then truly he becomes the help-seeker's slave. Similar considerations apply to the relationship between patients and physicians. If physicians cannot define their own rules – that is, when to help and in what ways – then they, too, are threatened with becoming the hostages of patients (or their representatives).

The typical cases of hysteria cited by Freud thus involved a *moral conflict* – a conflict about what the young women in question wanted to do with themselves. Did they want to prove that they were good daughters by taking care of their sick fathers? Or did they want to become independent of their elders, say, by having a family of their own, or in some other way? I believe it was the tension between these conflicting aspirations that was the crucial issue in these cases. The sexual problem – say, of the daughter's incestuous cravings for her father – was secondary (if that important); it was stimulated, perhaps, by the interpersonal situation in which the one had to attend to the other's body. Moreover, it was probably easier to admit the sexual problem to consciousness and to worry about it than to raise the ethical problem indicated. In the final analysis, the latter is a vastly difficult problem in living. It cannot be 'solved' by any particular manoeuvre but requires rather decision-making about basic goals, and, having made the decisions, dedicated efforts to attain them.

Some Remarks on Psychoanalysis and Ethics

The ethical values embodied in psychoanalysis derive from a number of sources: from the spirit of nineteenth-century science, from medicine, from certain philosophers (particularly Schopenhauer and Nietzsche), from Judaism and Catholicism, and, of course, from Freud himself (Bakan, 1959; Rieff, 1959). What are some of these values? The principal value is that knowledge, and especially self-knowledge, is good. This is the ethics of rationalism and science applied to the self as a part of nature. Integral to this ethic is also the belief that knowledge should be widely publicized and freely available. It must not be held secret by a small group and used as a source of power on its own behalf. Although in principle psychoanalysts espoused this scientific ethic, they betrayed it in practice as soon as they organized themselves into psychoanalytic groups.

Nor did Freud ever make explicit the moral values implicit in his theories and methods. What is the psychoanalytic view of a good human relationship – whether in marriage, friendship, business, or elsewhere? In vain do we search for answers in Freud's writings. One reason for this omission is that Freud liked to frame his investigations in the language of empirical – medical – studies. But *in the social sciences it is virtually impossible to conduct empirical studies wholly devoid of valuations.* This sort of physics is doomed to failure. Furthermore, it is easy to demonstrate that Freud and other psychiatrists favoured some values and opposed others. For example Freud not only 'discovered' infantile sexuality – he also advocated the sexual enlightenment of children; he not only studied the effects of sexual seductions on children – he also opposed this practice because he believed it was harmful to them.

When it came to paired human relations, Freud's position was that they are always based on the dominance of one partner and the submission of the other. He never discussed or advocated democracy, equality, reciprocity, or co-operation. His political beliefs were essentially Platonic – favouring an intellectual and moral elite which dictatorially governed the masses. Freud's misogynous utterances are well known (Freud, 1932). Probably less well appreciated is his insistence that the psychoanalytic relationship between analyst and analysand must be that of 'a 'superior and a subordinate' (Freud, 1914, p. 49). He did not seem to regard genuine co-operation between equals as either possible or desirable. To Freud, co-operation meant rather the imperfect person's wisdom to follow the leadership of a more accomplished superior.

In contrast to Freud, Adler (A. Adler, 1925; Ansbacher and Ansbacher, 1956) clearly articulated his concept of the morally desirable or 'mentally healthy' human relationship. It was characterized by a high degree of *social interest* and *co-operativeness*. He also stressed the values of truthfulness and competence while, at the same time, he placed less emphasis than Freud on self-knowledge.

Freud thus disguised and obscured, whereas Adler openly acknowledged and discussed, the moral values inherent in their respective psychological observations, theories, and therapies. I think this might be one of the reasons for the different receptions that Freudian and Adlerian psychologies received. Freud's work bore the stamp of the impartial, cool-headed natural scientist. It required the work of several scholars (Bakan, 1959; La Pierre, 1959; Rieff, 1959) to reveal and articulate the values inherent in Freudian psychology and psychotherapy. Adler, in contrast, did not conceal his values. Thus his work early diverged from medicine, psychology, and even from psychotherapy, and became closely associated with child-rearing, education, and social reform.

I suggested elsewhere (1957b) that certain aspects of the psychoanalytic procedure require a high degree of mutual co-operation between two relatively equal participants. By this I meant that although analyst and patient might be very unequal in regard to the possession of certain skills and the knowledge of how to apply them, they are, or should be, relatively equal in terms of power over each other.

From the evidence available – that is, judging from what psychoanalysts do and say – one could infer two almost antithetical ethical positions in regard to their practices. One would be that psychoanalysis favours a leader-follower, or domination-submission, type of human relationship; the other would be that the ethical value inherent in it is co-operation among equals. I believe that the aim of psychoanalytic therapy is, or should be, to maximize the patient's choices in the conduct of his life. This value must be entertained explicitly and must be espoused not only for him but potentially for everyone else as well. In other words, it is not the indiscriminate maximization of the patient's choices that is encouraged, for this could also be achieved by reducing the choices of others with whom he interacts (that is, by enslaving them). This, however, would run counter to the ethic of psychoanalysis, which favours increasing a person's choices by enhancing his knowledge and skills. In short, we should try to enrich our world through our own efforts, instead of merely seeming to enrich it by interfering with the efforts of our neighbour or by infringing on his rights and opportunities.

An Illustration of the Hysterical Game: Sullivan's 'Hysterical Dynamism'

Although Sullivan (1956) persisted in using many traditional psychiatric concepts, he employed the game model in his description of hysteria:

The hysteric might be said in principle to be a person who has a happy thought as to a way by which he can be *respectable* even though not living up to his *standards*. That way of describing the hysteric, however, is very misleading, for of course the hysteric never does have that thought. At least, it is practically *impossible to prove* that he has had that thought. ([Italics added] p. 203)

Sullivan here asserts that the hysteric is a person who impersonates respectability – in short, one who cheats. In the tradition of psychoanalysis, he adds that the hysteric does not do this consciously. While it does not seem that the hysteric carefully plans his strategy, it is a mistake to emphasize the unwitting quality of his behaviour. The question of precisely 'how conscious' a given mental act is has plagued psychoanalysis from its earliest days. I think this is largely a pseudo problem, for consciousness – or, self-reflective awareness – depends partly on the situation in which a person finds himself. In other words, it is partly a social characteristic, rather than simply a personal one.

In the following passage Sullivan provides an explicitly game-playing account of hysteria:

To illustrate how the hysteric dynamism comes into operation, let us say that a man with a strong hysterical predisposition has married, perhaps for money, and that his wife, thanks to his rather dramatic and exaggerated way of doing and saying things, cannot long remain in doubt that there was a very practical consideration in this marriage and cannot completely blind herself to a certain lack of importance that she has in her husband's eyes. *So she begins to get even*. She may for example, like someone I recently saw, develop a never-failing vaginismus, so that there is no more intercourse for him. And he will not ruminate on whether this vaginismus that is cutting off his satisfaction is directed against him, for the very simple reason that *if you view interpersonal phenomena with that degree of objectivity, you can't use an hysterical process to get rid of your own troubles*. So he won't consider that; but he will suffer terribly from privation and will go to rather extravagant lengths to overcome the vaginismus that is depriving him of satisfaction, the lengths being characterized by a certain rather theatrical attention to detail rather than deep scrutiny of his wife. But he fails again and again. Then one night when he is worn out, and perhaps has had a precocious ejaculation in his newest adventure in practical psychotherapy, he has the idea, 'My God, this thing is driving me crazy,' and goes to sleep . . .

Now the idea, 'This thing is driving me crazy,' is the *happy idea that I say the hysteric has*. He wakes up at some early hour in the morning, probably at the time when his wife is notoriously most soundly asleep, and he has a frightful attack of some kind. It could be literally almost anything, but it will be very impressive to anyone around. His wife will be awakened, very much frightened, and will call the doctor. But before the doctor gets there, the husband, with a fine sense of dramatic values, will let her know, in some indirect way, that he's terribly afraid he is losing his mind. She is reduced to a really agitated state by that. So when the doctor comes, the wife is in enough distress – in part because of whatever led to her vaginismus – to wonder if she might lose her own mind, and the husband is showing a good many odd symptoms. ([Italics added] pp. 204–6)

Sullivan's gift for portraying psychiatric 'diseases' as problems in living is beautifully demonstrated here. The mutually coercive relationship between husband and wife is especially noteworthy; and so is the patient's impersonating or taking the role of the mentally ill person.

Sullivan then proceeds to describe the 'hysterical dynamism' as a form of unconscious or inexplicit malingering without, however, using this term. He calls hysteria a form of 'inverted sublimation' – meaning that the patient 'finds a way of satisfying unacceptable impulses in a personally satisfactory way which exempts him from social blame and which thereby approaches sublimation. But the activity, if recognized, would not receive anything but social condemnation' (pp. 207–8). These remarks illustrate once again the use and function of non-verbal or indirect communications in hysteria, and also the close connection between hysteria and malingering. Phrased in terms of game-playing, the hysteric is here described as someone who would gladly take advantage of cheating if he believed he could get away with it. His cheating is so staged, moreover, as to lead those around him to interpret it not as a selfish stratagem but as un-avoidable suffering.

Another aspect of the game the hysteric plays – or of the sort of player he is, which, after all, determines the game he plays – may be discerned from the following passage:

The hysteric has a rather deep contempt for other people. I mean by this that he regards other people as comparatively shadowy figures that move around, I sometimes think, *as audience for his own perform-ance.* How does this show? Well – hysterics may be said to be the *greatest liars* to no purpose in the whole range of human personalities – nothing is good enough as it is. It always undergoes improvement in the telling; the hysteric simply has to exaggerate everything a little ... When they talk about their living – their interests, their fun, their sorrows and so on – only superlative terms will suffice them. And that, in a way, is a statement of the inadequacy of reality – which is what I mean when I say that hysterics are rather contemptuous of mere events and mere people. *They act as if they were accustomed to something better, and they are.* ([Italics added] pp. 209–10)

Sullivan here touches on the fact that the hysterical game is relatively unsophisticated. It is well suited to children, un-educated people, the oppressed, and the fearful; in brief, to those who feel that their chances for self-realization and success on their own are poor. Hence, they resort to impersonation and lying as strategies of self-advancement.

Most of the 'dynamisms' mentioned by Sullivan thus far illustrate the use of coercive manoeuvres. This is consistent with my thesis that hysteria is predominantly a coercive type of game.

Concerning hysterical conversion – that is, the use of iconic body signs – Sullivan writes:

Now, when there is this conversion, it performs a useful function; and that function occurs principally within the self-system . . . There one discovers sometimes the almost juvenilely simple type of operation set up to profit from the disabling system. The patient will often tell you in the most transparent fashion: 'If it were not for this malady then I could do –' and what follows is really quite a grandiose appraisal of one's possibilities. The disability functions as a convenient tool of security operations. (p. 216)

This, of course, is only one aspect of conversion, albeit a significant one. Sullivan's formulation is another way of saying that the hysteric plays at being sick because he is afraid that, if he tried to participate competently in certain real-life activities, he would fail. At the same time, by adopting this strategy the hysteric invites and assures his own defeat.

Sullivan's concluding remarks concerning hysteria strongly support the thesis that persons who tend to play this sort of game do so because they are impoverished in their game repertoire.

The presence of the hysteric dynamism as the outstanding way of meeting difficulties in living seems to me to imply that the patient has missed a good deal of life which should have been undergone if he was to have a well-rounded personality with a rather impressively good prospect for the future. *Because hysterics learn so early to get out of awkwardnesses and difficulties with a minimum of elaborate process*, life has been just as they sound: singularly, extravagantly simple. And so, even if one could brush aside the pathogenic or pathologic mechanisms, one would have persons who are not at all well-suited to complex interpersonal environment. There they just haven't had the experience; *they have missed out on an education that many other people have undergone*. ([Italics added] p. 228)

What a person considers worth doing or worth living for will depend on what he has learned. Whether coercive or co-operative games are preferred will necessarily vary with the person's attitude or taste. Accordingly, there may be those for whom playing the hysterical (or any other 'psychopathological') game is perfectly acceptable. There is a pervasive tendency in modern psychiatric theories and writings to disallow this possibility.[1]

[1] There is a striking resemblance in this regard between the psychoanalytic and classical Christian attitudes towards humanity. Neither accepts *people as people*! Psychoanalysis views and accepts people as generally 'sick' (i.e. 'neurotic' or 'psychotic'), whereas Christianity views and accepts them as generally 'sinful'.

Yet the facts of life seem to me to require that we explicitly recognize and accept a much greater diversity of human behaviour than we have heretofore.

Lying: A Specific Strategy in the Hysterical Game

It is considered anathema for a contemporary psychiatrist to speak of lying in connection with so-called mental illness. Once a person is called a 'patient', his psychiatrist is no longer permitted to consider such a thing as deception or mendacity. Anyone who speaks of lying in connection with psychiatric problems is immediately regarded as 'antipsychiatric' or 'antihumanitarian', meaning that he is both wrong and bad. This is regrettable, for it signifies the contemporary psychiatrist's sentimentalizing attitude towards the so-called mentally ill.

It has long been my impression that lying is one of the most significant phenomena in the field of psychiatry. In a sense, I am here restating one of Freud's earliest observations, namely, *that social hypocrisy is one of psychiatry's core problems.* He emphasized, for example, that both patients and physicians were in the habit of lying – if I may be permitted to reintroduce this useful word – when they spoke to each other about sex and money. How else are we to interpret Freud's story of his encounter with Chrobak in the case of the woman patient who was still a virgin after eighteen years of marriage? In relating this experience, Freud (1914, p. 296) noted that, as Chrobak saw it, the physician's social role and 'moral obligation' was to lie about the patient's condition, to protect the husband's reputation and the stability of the marriage. Whether to lie or not to lie were important issues in psychoanalysis from its very inception. Indeed, certain aspects of the psychoanalytic situation came into being in direct response to Freud's efforts to be forthright and truthful with his patients.

Adler, too, considered lying a significant subject for psychological investigation. This suggests that analysts were more candid in the early days of psychoanalysis than they are now in recognizing that people – including physicians and patients – often lied to each other. Evidently it is easier for a person to be observant about dishonesty if he feels that he has nothing to hide. Furthermore, the early psychoanalysts tended to avoid infantilizing patients. This is important, because the prototypal interaction in which one person lies to another is the parent–child situation: the parent does not tell the child the truth, but communicates rather what he considers to be 'good' for the child to hear. This paternalistic model of helpfulness by deception has had a powerful influence on nearly all human relationships.

In seventeenth-century Europe, for example, it was considered a compliment to be told that one could lie 'like a physician' (Fletcher, 1954, p. 42). Physicians were expected to treat patients as adults treated children. Hence it was not only justifiable but indeed required that one lie, since to tell patients painful truths was viewed as being unnecessarily cruel to them. This is still the prevailing medical ethic. Moreover, since psychoanalysis has become a respectable medical speciality, psychoanalysts too have turned away from scrutinizing the role of deceit in interpersonal relationships. Lying is either ignored or treated as something else – as amnesia, dissociative reaction, or whatnot.

Closely related to lying but not identical with it are mystification, obfuscation, and failure to clarify or explain. For example, a physician who avoids discussing the fee with a patient does not lie; he merely leaves something important unexplained and uncertain. The essential difference between lying and non-clarification is that in the latter case the speaker does not actively misinform; it is the same distinction as that between being misinformed and uninformed. However, by withholding information from a person who needs it, we may injure him just as much as if we lied to him.

A Clinical Illustration

The following observations are based on the psychoanalytic treatment of a young woman. I shall say nothing about why she came for help or what sort of person she was, but shall concentrate on only one aspect of her behaviour – namely, her lying. That she lied – in the sense that she communicated statement A to someone when she knew perfectly well that statement B was the truth

– became apparent early in the analysis and remained a crucial theme throughout it. The main reason she lied was that she conceived of herself as a trapped child confronted by an oppressive, unreasonable, and intrusive mother. The simplest and most effective way in which she could cope with her mother was by lying. Finding that her mother would accept her lies without openly challenging them encouraged her use of this strategy and firmly established lying as a characteristic feature of her personality. In her adult life, many of her friends and especially her husband ostensibly accepted her lies, much as her mother had. Her expectation in regard to her own untruthful communications was revealing. On the one hand, she hoped that her statements would be accepted as the truth; on the other hand, she wished that her lies would be challenged and unmasked. She realized that the price she paid for getting away with lying was *persistent psychological subservience* to those to whom she lied. I might add that this woman led a socially perfectly normal life and did not lie indiscriminately. She was inclined to lie only to people on whom she felt dependent or towards whom she felt angry. The more she valued a relationship, the more strongly convinced was she that she could not risk an open expression of personal differences, such as might result from a forthright exchange of conflicting needs or opinions.

In these situations of feeling trapped, lying became for this patient an indirect communication, similar to hysterical conversion or dream communication. As both she and I familiarized ourselves with the type of game she was playing, it became increasingly evident that the people to whom she lied knew, most of the time, that she was lying. And, of course, she did too. This did not in the least diminish the usefulness of the manoeuvre, the main value of which lay in *controlling the behaviour* (or response) of the other player(s). In terms of game-playing behaviour, it was as if she could not afford to take the chance to *play honestly*. Doing so would have meant that she had to make her move and then had to wait to see what her partner–opponent's move would be. The very thought of this made her unbearably anxious, especially when serious conflicts of interests between her and others were at stake. Hence, as against this type of 'open' game, she preferred to lie – that is, *to make communications whose effects she could foretell.* This protected her from the anxiety of not knowing what would happen. Thus, her marriage consisted of a complicated game of lies: her husband ostensibly accepted her lies as if they were truths and then used his knowledge that they were falsehoods to manipulate her in his own interests. This, then, gave her fresh ground for feeling oppressed and for lying to him.

Uncertainty and Control in Game-playing Behaviour

One of the characteristics of honest game-playing is that the moves of the other player(s) are predictable only within certain limits. For instance, in a game of chess or tennis one cannot foretell exactly – unless the players are very unevenly matched, in which case we can hardly speak of a 'game' at all – what one's opponent's move will be. To play a game, therefore, it is necessary to tolerate a measure – often a large measure – of uncertainty. This holds true also for the games of real-life social relationships. In other words, if a person plays honestly, he may often not be able to predict how others will react to him or to his efforts. Suppose, then, that for some reason it becomes very important to know, to be able accurately to control and predict, how another person will react to one's behaviour. This is the situation that is conducive to lying – and, more generally, to cheating – of a certain type. *The aim of the game now changes from task-orientation and task-mastery to the control of the other player's moves.* To be successful in this game, *information about the personality* of the other player(s) is essential; whereas for the game of task-mastery, what is needed is knowledge or skill.

These considerations have far-reaching implications for all situations in which those in authority are concerned with their subordinates' *personalities*, rather than with their *performances*. Psychiatric or psychologic reports on subordinates furnished to their superiors in various organizations, and the psychoanalytic training system, are illustrative examples (Szasz, 1958e). In these situations, and many others, the subordinate person's inadequate task-performance is often tolerated – indeed, is covertly encouraged – because the superior person has relinquished the value and goal of proficiency in a practical task and has adopted in its place the value of manipulating and 'treating' those under him.

In the case of chronic lying – for example, in a marriage relationship – it is clear that if this arrangement is acceptable to both parties, it provides an immense yield of rather cheaply earned security for them. This is accomplished through the *metacommunicative meanings* of the lie and its acceptance. By communicating a lie, the liar informs his partner that he is afraid of him and wishes to please him. This assures the recipient of the lie that he is in control of the liar and therefore need not be anxious about losing him; at the same time, he informs the liar that he, too, has an intense need for the relationship. By accepting the bribe of flattery and subservience implicit in being lied to, the recipient of the lie states, in effect, that he is willing to barter these items for the truth. Hence, the liar too is assured that he need not fear the loss of his object. The result is that both players in this game of mutual mendacity gain a measure – often a very large measure – of security.

As against this secure, though rather humiliating, arrangement a relationship based on the exchange of greater amounts of unmitigated truth is perhaps more vulnerable to dissolution. I think herein lies one of the reasons why some 'bad' marriages are much more 'stable' – that is, last longer – than many relatively 'good' ones. I use the terms 'bad' and 'good' here to refer to the presence or absence of such values as honesty, trustworthiness, dignity, and so forth. The continuation of a marriage or its dissolution by divorce, as mere facts, codify only the legal status of the relationships. They tell us nothing about the character of the marriage. This is the main reason why it is so foolish to regard an ongoing marriage as a sign of success in game-playing (e.g. 'mental health' or 'maturity'), and divorce as a sign of failure in it (e.g. 'mental illness' or 'immaturity'). Some marriages are actually defunct games; while divorce – which, in any case, forms an integral part of the marriage game – may represent the players' active participation in the game rather than their withdrawal from it.

A Summing Up

Viewed as a game, hysteria is characterized by the goal of domination and interpersonal control. The typical strategies employed in pursuing this goal are coercion by disability and illness. Deceitful gambits of various types, especially lies, also play a significant part in this game.

If we wish to address ourselves to the problem of the 'treatment' of hysteria (and of other 'mental illnesses'), we must first clearly face the question: In what directions – that is, towards what types of games – should the behaviour of the patient change? The word 'therapy' – in contrast to the word 'change' – implies that the patient's current behavioural state is 'bad' and that the direction in which the therapist wishes the patient to move is 'good', or at least 'better'. What is 'bad', 'better', and 'good' are here defined by the physician. Person-oriented psychotherapy requires, however, that patients be assisted in defining *their own conceptions of psychosocial 'illness' and 'health'*. This implies that a patient might set himself goals at variance with the values of his therapist: the patient may change in ways not specifically intended by the therapist, and indeed contrary to the therapist's personal preferences. In a sensible scheme of the psychotherapeutic interaction there must be room for this contingency.

Descriptions of therapeutic interventions and of modifications in patients' life activities might better be framed in terms of changes in the patients' game-orientations and strategies. In the case of the hysteric, for example, changes which might be labelled 'improvements' or 'cures' by some may occur in any one of the following directions: more effective coercion and domination of others; greater submission to others and increased preoccupation with suffering; withdrawal from the struggle over interpersonal control by progressive isolation from real-life relationships; and, finally, learning the goals and strategies of other games and becoming invested in some of them.

14 Object Relationships and the Game Model

Objects, Rules, and Games

In our effort to come together with our fellow man so that we can play the same game, we encounter two hindrances: one is the arduousness of learning; the other is the difficulty of forgetting. Perhaps this is another way of phrasing Freud's (1910a) classic formulation that the hysteric suffers from reminiscences (p. 16). In terms of object relationships, the hysteric suffers from the persistence of old (internal) objects and from his unmodified relationship to them. And in terms of the game model, the hysteric continues to play an old game, by outdated rules; and, unaware of doing so, he is gravely handicapped from relinquishing the game he is playing and developing an interest in new games.

Object Loss and Game Loss: Depression and Anomie

Let us compare object loss and depression on the one hand, with loss of social stability and anomie on the other. Some of the similarities between these phenomena rest on the similarities between groups and persons. As the individual needs supporting objects, and when he loses them becomes depressed – so, in this view, the group needs stable organizations, and when these crumble it develops *anomie* (De Grazia, 1948). The term 'anomie' was made popular by Durkheim, who meant by it the development of social apathy and disorganization as a result of a loss of previously valued goods and aspiration.

A great deal of psychiatric and sociological writing rests on the tacit assumption that loss of object and its vicissitudes characterize the frame of reference of personal conduct; and that loss of norms and the vicissitudes of anomie characterize the frame of reference of social conduct. What I want to suggest now is that norms and normlessness also affect the individual; that, in other words, *persons need not only other people but also rules worth following – or, more generally, games worth playing.*

It is perfectly clear that men suffer grievously when they can find no games worth playing, even though their object world might be quite intact. To account for this we must consider the relationship of the ego or self to games. Otherwise, we are forced to reduce all sorts of personal misery and suffering to considerations of object relationships. At the same time, we might regard the loss of game as another, more comprehensive, aspect of what has heretofore been called loss of object. Moreover, since the loss of a real or external object implies the loss of a player from the game – unless a perfect substitute for him can be found – such loss inevitably results in some changes in the game. It is evident, then, that 'players' and 'games' describe interdependent variables that together make up complex social systems – for example, families, organizations, societies, and so forth.

At this point, we might make still another connection between our present perspective and the traditional psychoanalytic view concerning the relationships between the personality and normative standards. In psychoanalysis, the ego ideal and the superego are the repositories of the rules and games that a person has learned, or has made for himself. The ego ideal is the set of rules to which the ego aspires. The superego – a term often used interchangeably with ego ideal – functions chiefly as a censor: 'This part [of the ego], which has the function (among others) of deciding which impulses are acceptable and which are not, is called the superego' (Fenichel, 1945, p. 18). The superego is said to be derived mainly from identification with the *frustrating* object. Thus, psychoanalysts speak of 'fatherly' and 'motherly' superegos (Fenichel, 1945, p. 104), depending on whether the father or mother was the disciplining parent. It is a mistake, however, to regard the superego as if it were entirely a censoring, prohibiting agency. Identifications with all types of parental and cultural values contribute to its formation. Prohibitions, permissions, and examples are all learned from other persons. Identifications with persons and roles, together with learning rules and games, make up the abstraction we call the 'personality'.

The connections between object and game outlined above may be illustrated by the following examples. A child that loses its mother loses not only an object – that is, a person invested with affection and other feelings – but is also precipitated into a human situation that constitutes a new game. The mother's absence means that other persons must care for some of the child's needs, and that he will henceforth have to relate to these persons.

Similar considerations hold for marriage. This game, traditionally conceived, lasts until death breaks it up. In so far as the players adhered to this rule, it provided them with great security against the trauma of game loss. It seems probable, indeed, that the institution of marriage has evolved – and has persisted as long as it has – not so much because it provides an ordered system of sexual relationships, nor because it is useful for child-rearing, but rather because it provides men and women with an extremely stable human relationship, in the context of a relatively unchanging game. Marriage has achieved this goal better than probably any other institution except the organized religions, which also tend to be very stable. This means that, having learned how to play these games, the person can stop learning and changing.

Loss of a parent in childhood, or loss of a spouse in adulthood, are situations in which loss of object and loss of game go hand in hand. There are other situations, however, in which loss of object and loss of game occur separately.

I shall briefly comment now on situations in which changes in games and object relationships occur asynchronously. Illustrative is the immigration of an entire family. In this case, especially if the immigrants are accompanied by friends and servants, we have a situation in which people have lost certain important games without having lost significant personal objects. Other factors which need not concern us here influence whether such circumstances soften or harden the blows of game loss. In general, such families either readily adapt themselves to new ways of living, a new language, and so forth – or go on living as if they never left home.

Instances in which object loss occurs unaccompanied by serious game loss illuminate the distinction between external and internal objects (Szasz, 1957a, p. 118). Changes in relation to external objects always result in changes in the game situation; whereas changes in relation to internal objects do not.

On Learning New Games

The concept of learning may be applied to a wide range of phenomena including skills, relations to objects, sign-using, rule-following, and game-playing. We can thus reinterpret certain key psychoanalytic concepts in terms of learning. Transference, for instance, could be viewed as a special case of 'playing an old game'. Indeed, in a recent paper Greenacre (1959) remarked: 'One thinks here of Fenichel's warning that *not joining in the game* is the principal task of handling the. transference'. ([Italics added] p. 488)

Although nowadays few analysts still believe that transference occurs only in the context of the psychoanalytic situation, many hold that this phenomenon pertains only to object relationships. I submit, however, that the characteristic features of transference can be observed in other situations as well, especially in the area of learned skills. For example, speaking a language with a foreign accent is similar to having a transference reaction. In the case of a transference reaction, one person behaves towards another as if the latter were someone else, previously familiar to him; moreover, the subject is usually unaware of the specific manifestations of his own transferred behaviour. In the same way, people who speak English (or some other language) with a foreign accent are generally unaware of their own distortions of it: to themselves, they sound as if they were speaking unaccented English; only when they hear their recorded voice, or when others point out, preferably by imitation, how they 'really sound' do they recognize their 'linguistic transferences'. The similarities here not only between the behavioural acts but also in the necessity for auxiliary channels of information (i.e. analyst, voice recording) are striking. This view of transference rests on empirical observations concerning the basic human tendency to generalize experiences.[1]

The developmental phase during which learning occurs, or from which a specific pattern of transference derives, is of crucial significance for its later modifiability. There are obvious limitations to unlearning one's earliest experiences – whether these relate to objects or to games. Such early learning is based on massive, indiscriminating identifications, and these identifications (internal objects) become an integral part of the personality. A far-reaching unlearning of these experiences may be virtually impossible. To aim for this goal may be unrealistic, and hence harmful. This does not mean that nothing can be done about such early impressions or about their effects on later personality functioning. On the contrary, only by properly recognizing the relatively unmodifiable aspects of one's personality can one discover and come to terms with oneself as a person. For example, it is virtually impossible for an adult to relinquish completely his mother tongue. Similar considerations apply to interest in sports. The persistence and stability of these behaviour patterns are significant for they may occur in spite of the immigrant's ready acquisition of other, more complex, games indigenous to the new cultural milieu.

On the other hand, experiences acquired in later life are usually learned discriminatingly and with only partial identifications. Learning of this type is unlearned much more readily than are 'motor rules' (Piaget, 1932) or so-called habits. Well-functioning new games may then replace older ones with hardly a trace of the past. If psychotherapists and patients fail to consider these facts concerning the modifiability of man, they risk trying to change what cannot be changed and failing to change what can.

The Polarities: Interest-Apathy, Hope-Anomie

Further connections between our knowledge of object relationships and game-playing behaviour may be sought by examining *attitudes* and *affects* from the perspective of the game model.

[1] A remarkably perceptive early formulation of this phenomenon was provided by Mach (1885), who called it the 'principle of continuity' (p. 57).

From the viewpoint of object relationship, 'being interested in' someone or something must be considered a fundamental affect. I refer here to the same sort of thing as what psychoanalysts call 'libidinal cathexis' or 'investment', or 'investment in objects'. From the standpoint of the experiencing person, objects may be said to exist only in so far as they are invested with interest. Morally, positive interest, such as love, is preferable to negative interest, such as hate; psychologically, either is preferable to loss of interest, such as apathy or indifference – for loss of interest threatens the very existence of the personality or self.

To live meaningfully, man must be interested and invested in more than just objects. He must have games he finds worth playing. The principal affective manifestations of an eagerness to engage in life are zest and hope and curiosity. As a loving attitude implies interest in persons – that is, in parents and children, wives and lovers, and friends – so a hopeful attitude implies interest in games, that is, in work and religion, contracts and institutions.

Hope, then, means an expectation of successful participation in a social interaction. This might imply winning, or playing well, or just enjoying what one is doing. The point is that a persistent interest in playing various games is a requirement of social living and of what is often thought of as 'mental health'. This is perhaps best revealed by the significance of work for the psychological integrity of modern man, especially when occupation is self-selected and is considered socially important. For people who do not possess inherited wealth and who must therefore work to earn a livelihood, doing a job constitutes one of the most important stable games. By remaining interested in working, men can avoid boredom and apathy on the one hand, and scrutiny of the self and its objects and games on the other. In other words, people who work could be said to 'play' the work-game, whereas the so-called idle rich 'work' at playing. For the latter, sports, travel, social gatherings, philanthropy, and other activities provide outlets for their need for games.

These remarks merely touch on the complicated subject of the relation between hope and religion. The essence of this problem is: what should man be *hopeful about*? In what should he *invest his hope*? Without pausing to try to answer or discuss these questions, I wish to emphasize only that investing hope in religious faith is perhaps one of the best psychological investments a person can make. This is because by investing a small amount of hope in religion – especially in a Christian religion – one gets back a great deal of it. After all, let us remember that religions *promise* gratifications and rewards of all sorts. Few other enterprises, other than fanatical nationalisms, promise as much. The rate of return on hope invested in religion is thus much higher than on hope invested in, say, rational work-a-day pursuits. Hence, those with small capitals of hope may do best by investing their 'savings' in religion.

It is clear, I think, that so long as a person lives and is not wholly unconscious, he has some sort of object relationships and is engaged in playing some kinds of games. Similarly, so long as man lives, he possesses some hope, however little. The Latin proverb, *Dum spiro, spero* – 'As long as I live (breathe), I hope' – asserted precisely this. The completely, utterly hopeless man, just as the completely objectless man, is a psychological impossibility.

Regression in Object Relationships and Game-playing

Different patterns of object relationships and of game-playing behaviour can be ordered according to a scale from the simple to the complex. In the case of object relationships, behaviour may range from mutually satisfying human interactions of great social complexity towards the upper end of the scale, to object relationships making use of non-human (substitute or 'part') objects towards the lower end of it. For game-playing behaviour, the range extends from technically complex, egalitarian games to serious degradations of rule-following and anomie. Yet, even in states of relatively profound normlessness, some patterns of rule-following remain discernible.

In his analysis of anomie, Merton (1957) illustrated the development of this condition by showing what happens when men dishonour the rules of the game and resort to cheating:

Thus, in competitive athletics, when the aim of victory is shorn of its institutional trappings and success becomes construed as 'winning the game' rather than 'winning under the rules of the game', a premium is implicitly set upon the use of illegitimate but technically efficient means. The star of the opposing football team is surreptitiously slugged; the wrestler incapacitates his opponent through ingenious but illicit techniques ... The emphasis on the goal has so attenuated the satisfactions deriving from sheer participation in the competitive activity that only a successful outcome provides gratification. Through the same process, tension generated by the desire to win in a poker game is relieved by successfully dealing one's self four aces or, when the cult of success has truly flowered, by sagaciously shuffling the cards in a game of solitaire. The faint twinge of uneasiness in the last instance and the surreptitious nature of public delicts indicate clearly that the institutional rules of the game are known to those who evade them. But cultural (or idiosyncratic) *exaggeration of the success-goal leads men to withdraw emotional support from the rules.* ([Italics added] pp. 135-6)

It is important to emphasize that cheating in a game betrays a measure of continued investment in and commitment to it. Evidently men cheat, among other reasons, because this is one way in which they can maximize their gains. But the things gained themselves have relevance, meaning, and value only in the context of the game. Illustrative is runaway inflation induced by a bankrupt government resorting to printing more money. Once it becomes widely apparent that the government has become a monopolistic enterprise at counterfeiting, money – as paper money – loses its value. It then becomes worth literally only as much as the paper on which it is printed. Soon, of course, it ceases to be called 'money'. Similar considerations apply to social games, whether they involve cheating in poker, tennis, science, marriage, or everyday living.

My point is that the degradations of game rules in so-called mental illnesses – for example, in hysteria, masochism, schizophrenia – can operate only so long as the patient's partner, and others around him, play the game according to rules other than, but complementary to, those by which the patient plays. If game stability in the degraded rules is to occur – that is, if the mental illness game is to remain stable even over a short span of time – the various players must *not* play the same game by the same rules. As a comic needs a straight man, so a schizophrenogenic parent needs a schizophrenic offspring, an agoraphobic wife a protective-controlling husband, and so forth. If the patient and the persons with whom he interacts were to play the same game by the same rules – that is, if they had a reciprocal or symmetrical relationship to one another – the mental illness game could not come into being and could not flourish.

These considerations are useful in formulating two very different strategies towards changing certain kinds of game-playing activity (such as conversion hysteria, paranoia, etc.). One is to fight fire with fire – that is, to adopt the same sorts of gambits as the patient uses. This is what Sullivan has advocated with the 'hysteric' (1956, pp. 219–20). Some of Rosen's (1953) strategies are also of this sort. Sometimes probably most psychotherapists – as well as persons in various walks of life – resort to this tactic. In the inflation analogy, this is what happens when enough people recognize the government as a massive counterfeiter and begin treating money as worthless: that is the end of at least that round of the inflation game.

In short, when all the players in a game throw the rules to the wind and devote themselves to cheating on a grand scale, the game becomes *rapidly self-liquidating*. Honestly played, egalitarian games on the other hand, tend to be *self-perpetuating*. They are potentially endless and are terminated either by death or by mutual consent.

The human cost of self-liquidating games is, of course, immense. Runaway inflation can last only a few months. Soon, money is completely worthless and the game is finished. A new game must then be started. The economic, moral, and social harm that has been wrought in this process of game-degradation and game-liquidation is staggering. Massive unemployment, anarchy and revolution are its usual aftermath. The same sort of consequences, though on a smaller scale, follow when hysterical or masochistic strategies are answered in kind. The 'patient's' 'mental illness' might be liquidated, but only at the cost of destroying the integrity, and often the very humanity, of one, or sometimes of all, of the participants in the game. The new game begun after the havoc is over is often on the level of a stereotyped living out of simple roles, awaiting release in death.

A fundamentally different strategy towards altering game-playing activities is entailed in psychoanalysis and some other forms of psychotherapy. In particular, the psychoanalytic situation may be regarded as a new game that therapist and patient undertake to play. It is a game different from all other games which the patient has been playing. It is, indeed, consciously constructed to be different from the patient's real-life games, since it is precisely this difference – codified in psychoanalysis as the contrast between 'transference' and 'reality' – that the patient is there to witness. In effect, then, the patient pays the analyst for a firsthand experience with a certain kind of game diversity, and specifically to be able to learn from it without incurring the usual penalties associated with trying out new games by actually playing them.

In short, psychoanalysis and psychoanalytic psychotherapy are learning situations in which an attempt is made to acquaint the player ('patient') more fully with the penalties of his own strategies ('neurosis'). Since he is usually not fully acquainted with these – and, on the contrary, tends to overrate the usefulness of his own game and underrate that of others – such an experience is often effective in arousing his desire to modify his behaviour. Once this desire is firmly established, the remainder – given a rational, searching, and intelligent effort at understanding and change by both patient and therapist – is relatively easy. It is easy – provided that the patient shares certain ethical aspirations inherent in this kind of psychotherapy. If he does not, the game he was playing might actually have been the best one for him. The effort to change it is then not likely to be 'therapeutic' for him, although it might help some persons around him.

Psychiatry as Social Action

The proposition that psychiatric operations constitute types of social action does not, I hope, require further proof. Although more obvious in the case of such interventions as involuntary mental hospitalization than in psychoanalysis, the idea that psychiatric activity of any sort is, among other things, a form of social action must be taken as our point of departure for what follows. I propose to distinguish three types of interventions, according to the psychiatrist's position vis-à-vis the games he encounters in his patients, their families, and the society in which they all live.

The psychiatrist as theoretical scientist is an expert on game-playing behaviour and shares his knowledge with those who hire him as an expert, or who wish to learn from him as a scientist who makes his knowledge public.

The psychiatrist as applied scientist or social engineer sorts out players and assigns them to the games which they can, or ought to, play.

The psychiatrist as social manipulator of human material punishes, coerces, or otherwise influences people to induce them to play, or to cease to play, certain games.

The first type of psychiatric activity is such as to make the work of the psychiatrist virtually indistinguishable from the work of the anthropologist, the historian, the social psychologist, the sociologist, or the so-called behavioural scientist. Psychiatry, so conceived, is a branch of social science. It must, nevertheless, remain of interest and significance to medicine, even if it ceases to parade as a biological science. For in so far as physicians try to help persons who are in distress – rather than *only* repair bodies that are deranged – they must have some familiarity with man as a social being.

The psychoanalytic therapist's social role, although not exactly that of a theoretical scientist, approximates to it. This is because his direct social impact is restricted to those who want to be exposed to it of their own volition. Psychoanalytic treatment cannot be forced on anyone; if it is, it is, in my opinion at least, not psychoanalysis.

The psychiatrist as social engineer, sorting out players for their 'proper' games, is encountered in the military services, marriage counselling, psychiatric hospitals, courts, and elsewhere (Szasz, 1956b, 1957e, 1959b). In the military services, for example, the psychiatrist's role is to determine who can play soldier and who cannot. Those who cannot are punished and/or released from the game. Similarly, in the state mental hospital, the psychiatrist's role is to separate the sane from the insane; to release the former and incarcerate the latter; and, in general, to assign those considered insane to playing the game of mental illness.

The third type of psychiatric intervention – the active manipulation of persons, families, groups, and so forth – is not clearly demarcated from the second type. The main distinction between the two is that in the former the psychiatrist's activity is limited, by and large, to sorting, classifying, or role-assigning, whereas in the latter it proceeds to moulding the 'patients' into the forms or roles that have been chosen for them. For instance, a psychiatrist who merely advises a married couple not to get a divorce classifies and sorts. He assigns the two individuals to the class of marriage partners. If, however, he does not stop there but proceeds to 'treat' both husband and wife, with the explicit aim of helping the marriage to succeed, then he also acts as a source of influence to bring about the desired role-playing in these individuals. Shock therapy, psychotherapy with children, and many other psychiatric interventions illustrate activities of this kind. The activities of the psychiatrist as social engineer, sorting people into the pigeonholes of 'identity' in which they 'belong' and making sure that they will fit by exerting the 'right' kinds of influence on them, have not passed unnoticed by some astute literary and philosophical observers (Dennis, 1955; Russell, 1953, 1954).

I think we ought to have very serious reservations about the second and third types of psychiatric activities. My much greater satisfaction with the first type of intervention does not, however, mean that I believe all is well with it. We ought to keep an open and critical mind towards it as well.

Conclusions

It is customary to define psychiatry as a medical speciality concerned with the study, diagnosis, and treatment of mental illnesses. This is a worthless and misleading definition. Mental illness is a myth. Psychiatrists are not concerned with mental illnesses and their treatments. In actual practice they deal with personal, social, and ethical problems in living.

I have argued that, today, the notion of a person 'having a mental illness' is scientifically crippling. It provides professional assent to a popular rationalization, namely, that problems of living experienced and expressed in terms of so-called psychiatric symptoms are basically similar to bodily diseases. Moreover, the concept of mental illness also undermines the principle of personal responsibility, the ground on which all free political institutions rest. For the individual, the notion of mental illness precludes an inquiring attitude towards his conflicts which his 'symptoms' at once conceal and reveal. For a society, it precludes regarding individuals as responsible persons and invites, instead, treating them as irresponsible patients.

Although powerful institutional forces lend their massive weight to the tradition of keeping psychiatric problems within the conceptual framework of medicine, the moral and scientific challenge is clear: we must recast and redefine the problem of 'mental illness' so that it may be encompassed in a morally explicit science of man. This, of course, would require a radical redivision of our ideas about 'psychopathology' and 'psychotherapy' – the former having to be conceived in terms of sign-using, rule-following, and game-playing, the latter in terms of human relationships and social arrangements promoting certain types of learning and values.

Human behaviour is fundamentally moral behaviour. Attempts to describe and alter such behaviour without, at the same time, coming to grips with the issue of ethical values are therefore doomed to failure. Hence, so long as the moral dimensions of psychiatric theories and therapies remain hidden and inexplicit, their scientific worth will be seriously limited. In the theory of personal conduct which I proposed – and in the theory of psychotherapy implicit in it – I tried to correct this defect by articulating the moral dimensions of human behaviours occurring in psychiatric contexts.

Epilogue

In Pirandello's play, *The Rules of the Game* (1919, p. 25), the following conversation takes place:

> Leone: Ah, Venanzi, it's a sad thing, when one has learnt every move in the game.
> Guido: What game?
> Leone: Why ... this one. The whole game – of life.
> Guido: Have you learnt it?
> Leone: Yes, a long time ago.

Leone's despair and resignation come from believing that there is such a thing as *the* game of life. Indeed, if mastery of *the* game of life were the problem of human existence, having achieved this task what would there be left to do? But there is no game of life, in the singular. The games are infinite.

Modern man seems to be faced with a choice between two basic alternatives. On the one hand, he may elect to despair over the lost usefulness or the rapid deterioration of games painfully learned. Skills acquired by diligent effort may prove to be inadequate for the task at hand almost as soon as one is ready to apply them. Many people cannot tolerate repeated disappointments of this kind. In desperation, they long for the security of stability – even if stability can be purchased only at the cost of personal enslavement. The other alternative is to rise to the challenge of the unceasing need to learn and relearn, and to try to meet this challenge successfully.

The momentous changes in contemporary social conditions clearly forewarn that – if man survives – his social relations, like his genetic constitution, will undergo increasingly rapid mutations. If this is true, it will be imperative that all people, rather than just a few, *learn how to learn*. I use the term 'to learn' rather broadly. It refers, first, to the adaptations that man must make to his environment. More specifically, man must learn the rules that govern life in the family, the group, and the society in which he lives. Further, there is the learning of technical skills, science, and learning to learn. Leone's problem is the dilemma of a man so far withdrawn from life that he fails to appreciate, and hence to participate in, the ever-changing game of life. The result is a shallow and constant life which may be encompassed and mastered with relative ease.

The common and pressing problem today is that, as social conditions undergo rapid change, men are called upon to alter their modes of living. Old games are constantly scrapped and new ones started. Most people are totally unprepared to shift from one type of game-playing to another. They learn one game or, at most, a few, and desire mainly the opportunity to live out life by playing the same game over and over again. But since human life is largely a social enterprise, social conditions may make it impossible to survive without greater flexibility in regard to patterns of personal conduct.

Perhaps the relationship between the modern psychotherapist and his patient is a beacon that ever-increasing numbers of men will find themselves forced to follow, lest they become spiritually enslaved or physically destroyed. By this I do not mean anything so naïve as to suggest that 'everyone needs to be psychoanalysed'. On the contrary, 'being psychoanalysed' – like *any* human experience – can itself constitute a form of enslavement and affords, especially in its contemporary institutionalized forms, no guarantee of enhanced self-knowledge and responsibility for either patient or therapist. By speaking of the modern psycho-therapeutic relationship as a beacon, I refer to a simpler but more fundamental notion than that implied in 'being psychoanalysed'. This is the notion of being a *student of human living*. Some require a personal instructor for this; others do not. Given the necessary wherewithal and ability to learn, success in this enterprise requires, above all else, the sincere desire to learn and to change. This incentive, in turn, is stimulated by hope of success. This is one of the main reasons why it is the scientist's and educator's solemn responsibility to clarify – never to obscure – problems and tasks.

I have tried to avoid the pitfalls of obscurantism which, by beclouding these problems, fosters discouragement and despair. We are all students in the metaphorical school of life. Here none of us can afford to become discouraged or despairing. And yet, in this school, religious cosmologies, nationalistic myths, and lately psychiatric theories have more often functioned as obscurantist teachers misleading the student than as genuine clarifiers helping him to help himself. Bad teachers are, of course, worse than no teachers at all. Against them, scepticism is our sole weapon.

Summary*

The principal arguments advanced in this book and their implications may be briefly summarized as follows.

1. Strictly speaking, disease or illness can affect only the body; hence, there can be no mental illness.

2. 'Mental illness' is a metaphor. Minds can be 'sick' only in the sense that jokes are 'sick' or economies are 'sick'.

3. Psychiatric diagnoses are stigmatizing labels, phrased to resemble diagnoses, and applied to persons whose behaviour annoys or offends others.

4. Those who suffer from and complain of their own behaviour are usually classified as 'neurotic'; those whose behaviour makes others suffer, and about whom others complain, are usually classified as 'psychotic'.

5. 'Mental illness' is not something a person *has*, but is something he *does* or *is*.

6. If there is no 'mental illness', there can be no 'hospitalization', 'treatment', or 'cure' for it. Of course, people may change their behaviour or personality, with or without psychiatric intervention. Such intervention is nowadays called 'treatment', and the change, if it proceeds in a direction approved by society, 'recovery', or 'cure'.

7. The introduction of psychiatric considerations into the administration of the criminal law – for example, the insanity plea and verdict, diagnoses of mental incompetence to stand trial, and so forth – corrupt the law and victimize the subject on whose behalf they are ostensibly employed.

8. Personal conduct is always rule-following, strategic, and meaningful. Patterns of interpersonal and social relations may be regarded and analysed as if they were games, the behaviour of the players being governed by explicit or tacit game rules.

9. In most types of voluntary psychotherapy, the therapist tries to elucidate the inexplicit game rules by which the client conducts himself; and to help the client scrutinize the goals and values of the life games he plays.

10. There is no medical, moral, or legal justification for involuntary psychiatric interventions, such as 'diagnosis', 'hospitalization', or 'treatment'. They are crimes against humanity.

* 1 January 1972

Bibliography

ADLER, A. (1907–37). Selections from his writings. In H. L. ANS-
BACHER and R. R. ANSBACHER (eds), *The Individual Psychology
of Alfred Adler*. New York: Basic Books, 1956.

ADLER, A. (1925). *The Practice and Theory of Individual Psychology*.
Translated by P. RADIN. Paterson, N.J.: Littlefield, Adams, 1959.

ADLER, A. (1931). *What Life Should Mean to You*. New York:
Capricorn Books, 1958.

ADLER, M. J. (1937). *What Man Has Made of Man. A Study of the
Consequences of Platonism and Positivism in Psychology*. New York:
Frederick Ungar, 1957.

ANSBACHER, H. L., and ANSBACHER, R. R. (eds) (1956). *The
Individual Psychology of Alfred Adler. A Systematic Presentation in
Selections from His Writings*. New York: Basic Books.

ARIETI, S. (1955). *Interpretation of Schizophrenia*. New York:
Robert Brunner.

ARIETI, S., and METH, J. M. (1959). 'Rare, Unclassifiable, Collective
and Exotic Psychotic Syndromes.' In S. ARIETI *et al.* (eds),
American Handbook of Psychiatry. Vol. I, Chapter 27, pp. 546–63.
New York: Basic Books.

BAKAN, D. (1959). *Sigmund Freud and The Jewish Mystical Tradition*.
Princeton, N.J.: Van Nostrand.

BIRDWHISTELL, R. L. (1959). 'Contribution of Linguistic-Kinesic
Studies to the Understanding of Schizophrenia.' In A. AUERBACK
(ed.), *Schizophrenia. An Integrated Approach*, Chapter 5, pp. 99–
124. New York: Ronald Press.

BRAITHWAITE, R. B. (1953). *Scientific Explanation. A Study of the
Function of Theory, Probability and Law in Science*. Based Upon
the Tarner Lectures, 1946. Cambridge: Cambridge University
Press, 1955.

BREUER, J., and FREUD, S. (1893–5). 'Studies on Hysteria.' In *The
Standard Edition of the Complete Psychological Works of Sigmund
Freud*. Vol. II. London: Hogarth Press, 1955.

BRIDGMAN, P. W. (1936). *The Nature of Physical Theory*. Princeton,
N.J.: Princeton University Press.

BRIDGMAN, P. W. (1959). *The Way Things Are*. Cambridge, Mass.:
Harvard University Press.

BURCHARD, E. M. L. (1960). 'Mystical and scientific aspects of the psychoanalytic theories of Freud, Adler and Jung.' *Amer. J. Psychotherapy*, *14:289*.

BURCKHARDT, J. (1868–71). *Force and Freedom*. New York: Meridian Books, 1955.

BUTLER, S. (1903). *The Way of All Flesh*. London: Penguin Books, 1953.

CHAPMAN, J. S. (1957). 'Peregrinating problem patients: Münchausen's syndrome.' *J.A.M.A.*, *165:927*.

COHEN, E. A. (1954). *Human Behaviour in the Concentration Camp*. Translated by M. H. BRAAKSMA. London: Jonathan Cape.

COLBY, K. M. (1955). *Energy and Structure in Psychoanalysis*. New York: Ronald Press.

CRITCHLEY, M. (1939). *The Language of Gesture*. London: Edward Arnold.

DE GRAZIA, S. (1948). *The Political Community. A Study of Anomie*. Chicago: The University of Chicago Press.

DENNIS, N. (1955). *Cards of Identity*. London: Weidenfeld and Nicolson.

DEUTSCH, H. (1942). 'Some forms of emotional disturbance and their relationship to schizophrenia.' *Psychoanalyt. Quart.*, *11*:301.

DEUTSCH, H. (1955). 'The impostor. Contribution to ego psychology of a type of psychopath.' *Psychoanalyt. Quart.*, *24*:483.

DOLLARD, J., and MILLER, N. E. (1950). *Personality and Psychotherapy. An Analysis in Terms of Learning, Thinking, and Culture*. New York: McGraw-Hill.

DOSTOEVSKY, F. M. (1861–2). *Memoirs from the House of the Dead*. Translated by JESSIE COULSON. New York: Oxford University Press, 1956.

EINSTEIN, A. (1933). 'On the Methods of Theoretical Physics.' In A. EINSTEIN. *The World as I See It*, pp. 30–40. New York: Covici, Friede, 1934.

EISSLER, K. R. (1951). 'Malingering.' In G. B. WILBUR and W. MUENSTERBERGER (eds). *Psychoanalysis and Culture*, pp. 218–53. New York: International Universities Press.

ENGELS, F. (1877). *Anti-Dühring*. Selection quoted in G. L. ABERNETHY (ed.). *The Idea of Equality. An Anthology*, pp. 196–200. Richmond, Va:. John Knox Press, 1959.

ERIKSON, E. H. (1950). *Childhood and Society*. New York: W. W. Norton.

FAIRBAIRN, W. R. D. (1952). *Psychoanalytic Studies of the Personality*. London: Tavistock Publications.

FAIRBAIRN, W. R. D. (1954). 'Observations on the nature of hysterical states.' *Brit. J. M. Psychol.*, *27*:105.

FENICHEL, O. (1945). *The Psychoanalytic Theory of Neurosis*. New York, W. W. Norton.

FERENCZI, S. (1912). 'To Whom Does One Relate One's Dreams?'

In S. FERENCZI. *Further Contributions to the Theory and Technique of Psycho-Analysis*, p. 349. London: Hogarth Press, 1950.

FERENCZI, S. (1916–17). 'Disease or Patho-neuroses.' In S. FERENCZI. *Further Contributions to the Theory and Technique of Psycho-Analysis*, pp. 78–89. London: Hogarth Press, 1950.

FIELD, M. G. (1957). *Doctor and Patient in Soviet Russia.* Cambridge, Mass.: Harvard University Press.

FLETCHER, J. (1954). *Morals and Medicine. The Moral Problems of: The Patient's Right to Know the Truth, Contraception, Artificial Insemination, Sterilization, Euthanasia.* Princeton, N.J.: Princeton University Press.

FREUD, S. (1893a). 'Charcot.' In *Collected Papers.* Vol. I, pp. 9–23. London: Hogarth Press, 1948.

FREUD, S. (1893b). 'Some Points in a Comparative Study of Organic and Hysterical Paralyses.' In *Collected Papers.* Vol. I, pp. 42–58. London: Hogarth Press, 1948.

FREUD, S. (1900). 'The Interpretation of Dreams' (I and II). In *The Standard Edition of the Complete Psychological Works of Sigmund Freud.* Vols IV and V, pp. 1–621. London: Hogarth Press, 1953.

FREUD, S. (1901). 'On Dreams.' In *The Standard Edition of the Complete Psychological Works of Sigmund Freud*, Vol. V, pp. 631–86. London: Hogarth Press, 1953. (Permission to reprint granted by W. W. Norton.)

FREUD, S. (1905a). 'Fragment of an Analysis of a Case of Hysteria.' In *The Standard Edition of the Complete Psychological Works of Sigmund Freud.* Vol. VII, pp. 1–122. London: Hogarth Press, 1953.

FREUD, S. (1905b). 'Three Essays on the Theory of Sexuality.' In *The Standard Edition of the Complete Psychological Works of Sigmund Freud.* Vol. VII, pp. 123–245. London: Hogarth Press, 1953.

FREUD, S. (1905c). 'Wit and Its Relation to the Unconscious.' In *The Basic Writings of Sigmund Freud*, pp. 633–803. Translated and edited, with an Introduction by A. A. BRILL. New York: Modern Library, 1938.

FREUD, S. (1909). 'General Remarks on Hysterical Attacks.' In *Collected Papers.* Vol. I, pp. 100–104. London: Hogarth Press, 1948.

FREUD, S. (1910a). 'Five Lectures on Psycho-Analysis.' In *The Standard Edition of the Complete Psychological Works of Sigmund Freud.* Vol. XI, pp. 1–55. London: Hogarth Press, 1957.

FREUD, S. (1910b). 'The Antithetical Sense of Primal Words. A Review of a Pamphlet by Karl Abel, *Über den Gegensinn der Urworte* (1884).' In *Collected Papers*, Vol. IV, pp. 184–91. London: Hogarth Press, 1948.

FREUD, S. (1913). 'Further Recommendations in the Technique of Psycho-Analysis.' In *Collected Papers.* Vol. II, pp. 342–65. London: Hogarth Press, 1948.

FREUD, S. (1914). 'On the History of the Psycho-Analytic Movement.' In *Collected Papers*. Vol. I, pp. 287–359. London: Hogarth Press, 1948.

FREUD, S. (1915). 'The Unconscious.' In *The Standard Edition of the Complete Psychological Works of Sigmund Freud*. Vol. XIV, pp. 159–204. London: Hogarth Press, 1957.

FREUD, S. (1916–17). *A General Introduction to Psychoanalysis*. Garden City, N.Y.: Garden City, 1943.

FREUD, S. (1920). 'Memorandum on the Electrical Treatment of War Neurotics.' In *The Standard Edition of the Complete Psychological Works of Sigmund Freud*. Vol. XVII, pp. 211–15. London: Hogarth Press, 1955.

FREUD, S. (1927). *The Future of an Illusion*. New York: Liveright, 1949.

FREUD, S. (1928). 'Dostoevsky and Parricide.' In *Collected Papers*. Vol. V, pp. 222–42. London: Hogarth Press, 1950.

FREUD, S. (1930). *Civilization and Its Discontents*. London: Hogarth Press, 1946.

FREUD, S. (1932). *New Introductory Lectures on Psycho-Analysis*. New York: W. W. Norton, 1933.

FREUD, S. (1940). *An Outline of Psychoanalysis*. New York: W. W. Norton.

FROMM, E. (1941). *Escape from Freedom*. New York: Rinehart.

FROMM, E. (1951). *The Forgotten Language. An Introduction to the Understanding of Dreams, Fairy Tales and Myths*. New York: Rinehart.

FROMM, E. (1955). *The Sane Society*. New York: Rinehart.

FROMM, E. (1957). 'Symbolic Language of Dreams.' In R. N. ANSHEN (ed.). *Language: An Enquiry into its Meaning and Function*. Chapter XII, pp. 188–200. New York: Harper.

FROMM, E. (1959). *Sigmund Freud's Mission: An Analysis of his Personality and Influence*. New York: Harper.

GALBRAITH, J. K. (1958). *The Affluent Society*. Boston: Houghton Mifflin.

GALLINEK, A. (1942). 'Psychogenic disorders and the civilization of the Middle Ages.' *Am J. Psychiat.*, 99:42.

GANSER, S. (1898). 'Über einen eigenartigen Hysterischen Dämmerzustand', *Arch. Psychiat.*, 30:633.

GLOVER, E. (1949). *Psychoanalysis*. London: Staples Press.

GOFFMAN, E. (1959). *The Presentation of Self in Everyday Life*. Garden City, N.Y.: Doubleday.

GOLDSTEIN, K. (1951). *Human Nature in the Light of Psychopathology*. Cambridge, Mass.: Harvard University Press.

GREENACRE, P. (1959). 'Certain technical problems in the transference relationship.' *J. Am. Psychoanalyt. A.*, 7:484.

GREGORY, R. L. (1953). 'On physical model explanations in psychology.' *Brit. J. Phil. Sc.*, 4:192.

GRODDECK, G. (1927). *The Book of the It: Psychoanalytic Letters to a Friend*. London: C. W. Daniel, 1935.

GRODDECK, G. (1934). *The World of Man, As Reflected in Art, in Words and in Disease*. London: C. W. Daniel.

GUILLAIN, G. (1959). *J.-M. Charcot, 1825–1893. His Life – His Work*. Edited and translated by PEARCE BAILEY. New York: Paul B. Hoeber.

HOLLINGSHEAD, A. B., and REDLICH, F. C. (1958). *Social Class and Mental Illness. A Community Study*. New York: John Wiley.

HORNEY, K. (1939). *New Ways in Psychoanalysis*. New York: W. W. Norton.

HUIZINGA, J. (1927). *The Waning of the Middle Ages*. New York: Doubleday, 1956.

HUXLEY, A. (1952). *The Devils of Loudun*. New York: Harper.

INKELES, A., and BAUER, R. A. (1959). *The Soviet Citizen. Daily Life in a Totalitarian Society*. Cambridge, Mass.: Harvard University Press.

JAKOBSON, R. (1957). 'The Cardinal Dichotomy in Language.' In R. N. ANSHEN (ed.). *Language: An Enquiry into its Meaning and Function*. Chap. IX, pp. 155–73. New York: Harper.

JESPERSON, O. (1905). *Growth and Structure of the English Language*. Ninth Edition. Garden City, N.Y.: Doubleday, 1955.

JONES, E. (1953, 1955, 1957). *The Life and Work of Sigmund Freud*. Vols 1, 2, 3. New York: Basic Books.

JUNG, C. G. (1940). *The Integration of the Personality*. Translated by STANLEY DELL. London: Routledge and Kegan Paul, 1952.

JUNG, C. G. (1945). *Psychological Reflections. An Anthology of the Writings of C. G. Jung*. Selected and edited by JOLANDE JACOBI. New York: Pantheon (Bollingen Series XXXI), 1953.

JUNG, C. G. (1952). *Symbols of Transformation. An Analysis of the Prelude to a Case of Schizophrenia*. Translated by R. F. C. HULL. New York: Pantheon (Bollingen Series XX), 1956.

KRÄMER, H., and SPRENGER, J. (1486). *Malleus Maleficarum*. Translated, with an Introduction, Bibliography and Notes by the REV. MONTAGUE SUMMERS. London: Pushkin Press, 1948.

LANGER, S. K. (1942). *Philosophy in a New Key*. Cambridge, Mass.: Harvard University Press. (Page references to Mentor Books edition, 1953.)

LAPIERRE, R. (1959). *The Freudian Ethic*. New York: Duell, Sloan and Pearce.

LEWINSOHN, R. (1958). *A History of Sexual Customs*. Translated by ALEXANDER MAYCE. New York: Harper.

LINCOLN, A. (1858). From a letter in C. MORLEY and L. D. EVERETT (eds). *Familiar Quotations*, p. 455. Boston: Little, Brown, 1951.

MACINTYRE, A. C. (1958). *The Unconscious. A Conceptual Analysis*. London: Routledge & Kegan Paul.

MACH, E. (1885). *The Analysis of Sensations and the Relation of the Physical to the Psychical*. Translated by C. M. WILLIAMS. Revised and supplemented from the Fifth German Edition by SYDNEY WATERLOW, with a new Introduction by THOMAS S. SZASZ. New York: Dover Publications, 1959.

MANN, T. (1954). *Confessions of Felix Krull: Confidence Man*. Translated by DENVER LINDLEY. New York: Knopf, 1955.

MARX, K. (1844). 'A Critique of the Hegelian Philosophy of Right.' In K. MARX. *Selected Essays*, pp. 11–39. Translated by H. J. STENNING. New York: International Publishers, 1926.

MAURER, D. W. (1940). *The Big Con, The Story of the Confidence Man and the Confidence Game*. Indianapolis: Bobbs-Merrill.

MEAD, G. H. (1934). *Mind, Self and Society. From the Standpoint of a Social Behaviorist*. Edited, with an Introduction, by CHARLES W. MORRIS. Chicago: the University of Chicago Press.

MEERLOO, J. A. M. (1955). 'Medication into submission, the danger of therapeutic coercion.' *J. Nerv. & Ment. Dis.*, *122*:353.

MEERLOO, J. A. M. (1956). *The Rape of the Mind. The Psychology of Thought Control*. New York: World.

MENNINGER, K. A. (1938). *Man Against Himself*. New York: Harcourt, Brace.

MERTON, R. K. (1957a). *Social Theory and Social Structure*. Revised and enlarged edition. Glencoe, Ill.: The Free Press.

MILLER, N. E., and DOLLARD, J. (1941). *Social Learning and Imitation*. New Haven: Yale University Press.

MISES, R. VON (1951). *Positivism. A Study in Human Understanding*. New York: George Braziller, 1956.

MONTAGU, A. (1953). *The Natural Superiority of Women*. New York: Macmillan.

MORRIS, C. W. (1946). *Signs, Language and Behavior*. New York: Prentice-Hall.

MORRIS, C. W. (1955). 'Foundations of the Theory of Signs.' In O. NEURATH, R. CARNAP, and C. W. MORRIS (eds). *International Encyclopedia of Unified Science*, Vol. I, pp. 77–137. Chicago: the University of Chicago Press.

MUNTHE, A. (1930). *The Story of San Michele*. New York: Dutton.

NADEL, S. F. (1954). *Nupe Religion*. Glencoe, Ill.: The Free Press.

NOYES, A. P. (1956). *Modern Clinical Psychiatry*. Fourth edition. Philadelphia: W. B. Saunders.

PARRINDER, G. (1958). *Witchcraft*. London: Penguin Books.

PARSONS, T. (1952). *The Social System*. Glencoe, Ill.: The Free Press.

PARSONS, T. (1958a). 'Definitions of Health and Illness in the Light of American Values and Social Structure.' In E. G. JACO (ed.). *Patients, Physicians and Illness*. Chapter 20, pp. 165–87. Glencoe, Ill.: The Free Press.

PARSONS, T. (1958b). 'Social structure and the development of the personality.' Freud's contribution to the integration of psychology and sociology. *Psychiatry*, *21*:321.

PAULING, L. (1956). 'The molecular basis of genetics.' *Am. J. Psychiat.*, *113*:492.

PETERS, R. S. (1958). *The Concept of Motivation*. London: Routledge & Kegan Paul.

PIAGET, J. (1928). *Judgment and Reasoning in the Child*. Translated by MARJORIE WARDEN. London: Routledge & Kegan Paul, 1952.

PIAGET, J. (1932). *The Moral Judgment of the Child*. Translated by MARJORIE GABAIN. Glencoe, Ill.: The Free Press.

PIAGET, J. (1951). *Play, Dreams and Imitation in Childhood*. Translated by C. GATTEGNO and F. M. HODGSON. London: William Heinemann.

PIAGET, J. (1952a). *The Child's Conception of Number*. Translated by C. GATTEGNO and F. M. HODGSON. London: Routledge & Kegan Paul.

PIAGET, J. (1952b). *The Origins of Intelligence in Children*. Translated by MARGARET COOK. New York: International Universities Press.

PIAGET, J. (1953). *Logic and Psychology*. With an Introduction on Piaget's Logic by W. MAYS. Manchester: The University Press.

PIAGET, J. (1954). *The Construction of Reality in the Child*. Translated by MARGARET COOK. New York: Basic Books.

PIRANDELLO, L. (1919). 'The Rules of the Game.' Translated by ROBERT RIETTY. In L. PIRANDELLO: *Three Plays*. Introduced and edited by E. MARTIN BROWNE. London: Penguin Books, 1959.

POPPER, K. R. (1944–5). *The Poverty of Historicism*. Boston: Beacon Press, 1957.

POPPER, K. R. (1945). *The Open Society and Its Enemies*. Princeton, N.J.: Princeton University Press, 1950.

POPPER, K. R. (1957). 'Philosophy of Science: A Personal Report.' In C. A. MACE (ed.). *British Philosophy in the Mid-Century*, pp. 153–91. New York: Macmillan.

PURTELL, J. J., ROBINS, E., and COHEN, M. E. (1951). 'Observations on clinical aspects of hysteria.' *J.A.M.A.*, *146*:902.

RAPOPORT, A. (1954). *Operational Philosophy : Integrating Knowledge and Action*. New York: Harper.

REICHENBACH, H. (1947). *Elements of Symbolic Logic*. New York: Macmillan.

REICHENBACH, H. (1951). *The Rise of Scientific Philosophy*. Berkeley: University of California Press.

RIEFF, P. (1959). *Freud, The Mind of the Moralist*. New York: Viking.

ROHEIM, G. (1943). *The Origin and Function of Culture*. Nervous and Mental Disease Monograph No. 69. New York: Nervous and Mental Disease Monographs.

Rosen, J. N. (1953). *Direct Analysis: Selected Papers*. New York: Grune & Stratton.

Ruesch, J. (1959). 'General Theory of Communication in Psychiatry'. In S. Arieti *et al.* (eds.). *American Handbook of Psychiatry*. Vol. I, Chapter 45, pp. 895–908. New York: Basic Books.

Ruesch, J., and Bateson, G. (1951). *Communication. The Social Matrix of Psychiatry*. New York: W. W. Norton.

Russell, B. (1922). Introduction to L. Wittgenstein's *Tractatus Logico-Philosophicus*, pp. 7–8. London: Routledge & Kegan Paul.

Russell, B. (1945). *A History of Western Philosophy*. New York: Simon and Schuster.

Russell, B. (1948). *Human Knowledge: Its Scope and Limits*. New York: Simon and Schuster.

Russell, B. (1953). 'Satan in the Suburbs, or Horrors Manufactured Here.' In B. Russell. *Satan in the Suburbs and Other Stories*, pp. 1–59. New York: Simon and Schuster.

Russell, B. (1954). 'A Psychoanalyst's Nightmare: Adjustment – A Fugue.' In B. Russell. *Nightmares of Eminent Persons*, pp. 21–30. London: Bodley Head.

Ryle, G. (1949). *The Concept of Mind*. London: Hutchinson's University Library.

Schiller, J. C. F. (1798). 'Der Ring des Polykrates.' In Schiller. *Werke*. Vol. I, pp. 176–9. 12 Vols. Mit Einleitung von Gotthilf Lachenmaier. Berlin-Leipzig: Th. Knaur Nacht, 1908.

Schlauch, M. (1942). *The Gift of Language*. New York: Dover, 1955.

Strachey, J. (1934). 'The nature of the therapeutic action of psychoanalysis.' *Internat. J. Psycho-Analysis*, *15*:127.

Sullivan, H. S. (1947). *Conceptions of Modern Psychiatry*. The First William Alanson White Memorial Lecture. Washington, D.C.: the William Alanson White Psychiatric Foundation.

Sullivan, H. S. (1953). *The Interpersonal Theory of Psychiatry*. Edited by H. S. Perry and M. L. Gawel. With an Introduction by M. B. Cohen. New York: W. W. Norton.

Sullivan, H. S. (1956). *Clinical Studies in Psychiatry*. Edited by H. S. Perry, M. L. Gawel, and M. Gibbon. With a Foreword by D. M. Bullard. New York: W. W. Norton.

Szasz, T. S. (1956a). 'Some observations on the relationship between psychiatry and the law.' *A.M.A. Arch. Neurol. & Psychiat.*, *75*:297.

Szasz, T. S. (1956b). 'Malingering: "Diagnosis" or social condemnation? Analysis of the meaning of "diagnosis" in the light of some interrelations of social structure, value judgment, and the physician's role.' *A.M.A. Arch. Neurol. & Psychiat.*, *76*:432.

Szasz, T. S. (1956c). 'On the experiences of the analyst in the psychoanalytic situation. A contribution to the theory of psychoanalytic treatment.' *J. Am. Psychoanalyt. A.*, *4*:197.

SZASZ, T. S. (1957a). *Pain and Pleasure. A Study of Bodily Feelings.* New York: Basic Books.

SZASZ, T. S. (1957b). 'On the theory of psycho-analytic treatment. *Internat. J. Psycho-Analysis, 38*:166.

SZASZ, T. S. (1957c). 'A contribution to the psychology of schizophrenia.' *A.M.A. Arch. Neurol. & Psychiat., 77*:420.

SZASZ, T. S. (1957d). 'Commitment of the mentally ill: "Treatment" or social restraint?' *J. Nerv. & Ment. Dis., 125*:293.

SZASZ, T. S. (1957e). 'Psychiatric expert testimony: its covert meaning and social function.' *Psychiatry, 20*:313.

SZASZ, T. S. (1958a). 'Psychoanalysis as method and as theory.' *Psychoanalyst. Quart., 27*:89.

SZASZ, T. S. (1958b). 'Psychiatry, ethics, and the criminal law.' *Columbia Law Review, 58*:183.

SZASZ, T. S. (1958c). 'Scientific method and social role in medicine and psychiatry.' *A.M.A. Arch. Int. Med., 101*:228.

SZASZ, T. S. (1958d). 'Men and machines.' *Brit. J. Phil. Sci., 8*:310.

SZASZ, T. S. (1958e). 'Psycho-analytic training: a sociopsychological analysis of its history and present status.' *Internat. J. Psycho-Analysis, 39*:598.

SZASZ, T. S. (1958f). 'Politics and mental health: some remarks apropos of the case of Mr Ezra Pound.' *Am. J. Psychiat. 115*:508.

SZASZ, T. S. (1959a). 'A Critical Analysis of Some Aspects of the Libido Theory: The Concepts of Libidinial Zones, Aims, and Modes of Gratification.' In L. BELLAR (cons. ed.). *Conceptual and Methodological Problems in Psychoanalysis. Ann. N.Y. Acad. Sc., 76*:975.

SZASZ, T. S. (1959b). 'The classification of "mental illness". A situational analysis of psychiatric operations.' *Psychiat. Quart., 33*:77.

SZASZ, T. S. (1959c). 'Recollections of a Psychoanalytic Psychotherapy: the Case of the "Prisoner K".' In A. BURTON (ed.). *Case Studies in Counseling and Psychotherapy.* Chapter 4, pp. 75–110. Englewood Cliffs, N.J.: Prentice-Hall.

SZASZ, T. S. (1959b). 'Psychoanalysis and Medicine.' In M. LEVITT (ed.). *Readings in Psychoanalytic Psychology.* Chapter 24, pp. 355–74. New York: Appleton-Century-Crofts.

SZASZ, T. S. (1959e). 'Language and Pain' In S. ARIETI *et al.* (eds). *American Handbook of Psychiatry.* Vol. I, Chapter 49, pp. 982–99. New York: Basic Books.

SZASZ, T. S. (1959f). 'The communication of distress between child and parent.' *Brit. J. Med. Psychol., 32*:161.

SZASZ, T. S. (1959g). 'Psychiatry, psychotherapy, and psychology.' *A.M.A. Arch. Gen. Psychiat., 1*:455.

SZASZ, T. S. (1960a). 'Mach and psychoanalysis.' *J. Nerv. & Ment. Dis., 130*:6.

SZASZ, T. S. (1960b). 'The myth of mental illness.' *American Psychologist*, *15*: 113.

SZASZ, T. S. (1960c). 'Moral conflict and psychiatry.' *Yale Rev.*, *49*: 555.

SZASZ, T. S. (1960d). 'Civil liberties and the mentally ill.' *Cleveland-Marshall Law Rev.* *9*: 399.

SZASZ, T. S., and HOLLENDER, M. H. (1956). 'A contribution to the philosophy of medicine. The basic models of the doctor–patient relationship.' *A.M.A. Arch. Int. Med.*, *97*: 585.

VAIHINGER, H. (1911). *The Philosophy of 'As If.' A System of the Theoretical, Practical, and Religious Fictions of Mankind*. Translated by C. K. OGDEN. London: Routledge & Kegan Paul, 1952.

VON DOMARUS, E. (1944). 'The Specific Laws of Logic in Schizophrenia.' In J. S. Kasanin (ed.). *Language and Thought in Schizophrenia*, pp. 104–14. Berkeley and Los Angeles: University of California Press.

WEINBERG, J. R. (1950). *An Examination of Logical Positivism*. London: Routledge & Kegan Paul.

WEINER, H., and BRAIMAN, A. (1955). The Ganser syndrome: a review and addition of some unusual cases. *Am. J. Psychiat.*, *111*: 767.

WERTHAM, F. (1949). *The Show of Violence*. Garden City, N.Y.: Doubleday & Co.

WHITEHEAD, A. N., and RUSSELL, B. (1910). *Principia Mathematica*. Second edition, Vol. I. Cambridge University Press. 1950.

WOODGER, J. H. (1952). *Biology and Language. An Introduction to the Methodology of the Biological Sciences Including Medicine*. Cambridge: Cambridge University Press.

WOODGER, J. H. (1956). *Physics, Psychology and Medicine. A Methodological Essay*. Cambridge: Cambridge University Press.

ZIEGLER, F. J., IMBODEN, J. B., and MEYER, E. (1960). 'Contemporary conversion reactions: a clinical study.' *Am. J. Psychiat.*, *116*: 901.

ZILBOORG, G. (1935). *The Medical Man and the Witch During the Renaissance*. The Hideyo Nogushi Lectures. Baltimore: Johns Hopkins Press.

ZILBOORG, G. (1941). *A History of Medical Psychology*. In collaboration with G. W. HENRY. New York: W. W. Norton.

ZILBOORG, G. (1943). *Mind, Medicine, and Man*. New York: Harcourt, Brace.

Index

Index

Psychosis, 103, 126, 238; *see also* Schizophrenia
Psychosocial laws, 23
Psychosocial method, 46
Psychosomatic symptoms, 100
Psychotherapy, 73, 74–5, 131–2, 235, 255, 260, 264–7, 272; *see also* Psychoanalytic treatment
Public school teacher (U.S.A.) and Soviet physician, 77
Purtell, J. J., 104

Rapoport, A., 128, 133–4
Reclassification, of behaviour, 55–8, 126–7
Redlich, F. C., 75
Referral system, 88
Regression, 137
  vs. in fantilization, 170–2
  in object relationships, 262–5
Reichenbach, H., 111, 121, 124, 125
Religion, 23, 30, 138, 165, 182–3
  and hope, 261–2
  and oppression, 183–5
  see also Biblical rules
Representation, of objects, 61–4
Rieff, P., 244, 245
Roheim, G., 176
Role-taking, 29, 161–2; *see also* Helpfulness, Helplessness, Impersonation, Learning
Roles, 29, 161–2, 232–8; *see also* Helpfulness, Helplessness, Impersonation, Learning
Rosen, J. N., 264
Rule-consciousness, 210
Rule-following, *see* Behaviour
Rules, classification of, 164–8
  morals and superego, 159–63
  see also Behaviour
Rules of the Game, The (Pirandello), 271
Russell, B., 94, 113, 128, 186, 267
Ryle, G., 99

Saltpêtrière, 37, 40, 47, 124
Scapegoat theory of witchcraft, 193–9
Schiller, J. C. F., 179
Schizophrenia, 50, 69, 112, 124, 125, 138, 228, 263
Schizophrenic bodily symptoms, as non-discursive language, 138
Schizophrenic 'thought disorder', 50
Scientism, 201
Schlauch, M., 129
Schopenhauer, A., 244
Secondary gain, 140, 207–8
Secondary process, 116
Self-help, 212
  in hysteria, 239–42
Self-protection, 146
Semantics, 121
Semiotic, 20
Sermon on the Mount, The, 181
Shakespeare, W., 31
Sign-using, 23, 25, 27–9; *see also* Behaviour, Language
Signs, concept of, 111
  psychiatry as study of, 64
  see also Communications, Conventional signs, Iconic signs, Indexical signs
Simulation of illness, *see* Malingering
Slave psychology, 180
Social action, psychiatry as, 265–7
Social conditions, *see* Therapeutic situation
Social control, medical care as, 81–5
Social interest, 245
Social reform, 42
Social rules, 165, 166
Social worker (U.S.A.) and Soviet physician, 77, 81
Society, closed *vs.* open, 23
Sociology, 20, 24, 156, 174–7
  and biology, 158–9